Birth Writes

A Collection of Real Life Birth Stories

Edited by Carole Monnier Clark
with Chelsie Anderson

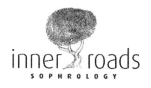

inner roads
SOPHROLOGY

The Live with Positivity Series

Birth Writes: A Collection of Real Life Birth Stories

ISBN: 978-1-5262-0659-6

Copyright ©2016 Carole Monnier Clark
Interior design by Lizzie Harwood at editordeluxe.com
Cover design by Verónica Cyrot Natera
Copyedited by Laura Slavik Fortin

Published by
Inner Roads Sophrology: The Live with Positivity Series

For my daughters, Liliane and Mira

Contents

A Note from the Editors

Many years ago, we shared our birth stories with each other while we tended to our newborns in a cozy living room during the long Canadian winter. We quickly realized that we craved more, but weren't sure where to find stories told by diverse voices sharing their raw experiences of labour and delivery as it happens today. The next step seemed obvious.

From the first call to submissions, that's exactly what this project has done. The stories included in this collection are as unique one from the other as the families who experienced them, all the while offering truths that will resonate with those who read them.

Between these covers you'll find heart-stoppers, tear-jerkers, laugh-out loud and ah-ha! moments, while running the gauntlet of birth experiences as varied and unpredictable as birth itself.

By sharing this collection of twenty-one stories the aim is to initiate a dialogue for women and their partners surrounding birth, a universal and deeply humanizing experience, while creating a community of support for families through the telling and sharing of birth stories.

We hope that you take away as much enjoyment, inspiration and healing from these stories as we have.

—Carole & Chelsie

Having Ahna at Home
by Heather Rader

"Can we come visit you in the hospital?" my fifth-grade students asked.

"I'm having my baby at home, not the hospital," I said.

"Can you do that? Are you allowed? What about when the doctor has to pull out the baby? What about the medicine in your back?"

I answered the questions one at a time. "Yes, I'm allowed. Many women choose to have their babies at home. I will have midwives with me whose job it is to care for moms and babies. You don't need any medicine to be able to deliver a baby. Not in your back, not anywhere."

"But why?"

"Because I choose to."

When I think back to the birth of my first child, I remember the fives. My water broke at 5:00 a.m. My baby was five weeks early. My husband followed the ambulance to the hospital at eighty-five miles per hour. My son weighed 5 pounds, 5 ounces at birth. Jamin Kurtis's tiny, star-like hands had five fingers each. I counted before they whisked him away.

In the NICU I had to show identification and scrub like a surgeon. I remember the thick IV lines in Jamin's hands, wrapped with tape to hold them in. The leads for the vital-signs monitors tracking his heart and chest wall movement covered his entire abdomen. A nasal C-PAP (Continuous Positive Airway Pressure) providing supplemental oxygen through his nose was taped to his face. A gavage, a feeding tube going down to his stomach, delivered my milk. He was beautiful and seemed very, very tiny in contrast to the technology surrounding him. This was not what I had expected.

I relived that birth in both my waking and sleeping hours: lonely ride in the ambulance, unfamiliar hospital and staff, large episiotomy, hemorrhaging after birth, and watching my baby being taken away. My husband Kurt and I appreciated those tubes that brought him food and oxygen, but it was a white-knuckle experience, not the birth story I had planned. A few months later it was discovered that I had a genetic disorder known as Celiac Sprue that, in addition to damaging my digestive system, brought many other complications, including anemia, which was the likely cause of my son's early exit.

Two years later we conceived another child and I got in touch with fear. Every twinge, each cramp, all the pain brought me back to, "Will I have her early, too?" During my third trimester, I took my students on a field trip and, in the back of a bouncy school bus, I started having contractions. It was too early; eight weeks too early. At my appointment, the doctor confirmed that my cervix had begun to efface and dilate slightly, which could be normal for a second pregnancy. Not wanting to take any chances, I was admitted to the hospital with irregular but persistent contractions, where I received a shot of steroids for my baby's lungs, should she come early. For the next nineteen days, I was to take terbutaline every four hours and be on complete bed rest. The nurse said taking the medication would feel like several shots of espresso. What she didn't say was that I would spend the next three weeks on my left side in a heart-racing, paranoid, sleep-deprived stupor.

I waited and waited for that early baby, but instead I was induced three days after my due date. The induction required that I labour in bed, most of the time on my back. As I entered the second stage of labour, the staff coached me to "*Push!* On the count of three!" and I burst a blood vessel in my eye. Again, I had an episiotomy. My recovery was much quicker this time, but for several days I felt (and looked) like a losing boxer. Our daughter Maya was 8 pounds of pink, active, healthy baby. Why had we been so fearful? I wondered if either of us had ever been in any real danger requiring the interventions.

While doctors and hospitals had been necessary for our son, we realized the extent to which hospital procedures had contributed to our anxiety and inability to experience joy with our daughter.

When we conceived a third time, we decided to do it our way. We believed that pregnancy was natural, normal, and safe. I believed my body would know how to carry a baby to term and give birth, if only I could get my mind out of the way. At thirty-two weeks the contractions started again. This time, after a fetal fibronectin test and exam reassured us that I was not progressing too rapidly, I was treated with water, rest, herbal tinctures (cramp bark and motherwort) and the elimination of dairy products from my diet. The contractions ceased, and I was able to continue working. My midwife, Marijke, told me, "If your baby comes early, it is because she will do better on the outside than the inside. I think you are going to carry this baby to term, but your body knows what it's doing." I felt empowered and supported, no matter what the outcome.

My due date passed. I began walking a couple miles a day and writing my birth affirmation over and over. *I am open to the joy. I am ready to experience a healthy birth through a smooth, positive, productive labour at home and trust the rhythms of my body. My baby will be born anterior, pink, radiant, alert, and healthful; she will be a natural nurser.* Turbulent emotions washed over me. Some mornings I would wake feeling strong and miraculous, only to find myself fearful and sobbing an hour later. One day a friend telephoned and said: "I just had to call. Two home births came into the ER last night, dead on arrival. The nurse said if they had been delivered in the hospital they would've been all right."

Dead on arrival. I was stunned that this longtime friend would share such news with me so close to delivering my baby at home. After some reflection, I realized that it was her fear speaking to me, not real dangers. In fact, she represented what many people believe: that home birth is risky. But my pregnancy was not high risk, and I did not want the hospital surroundings. I wanted my bed, birth tub, exercise ball, husband, bathroom, food and family. I didn't want to labour in bed with handles or buttons or give birth on my back in the worst possible position for my pelvis. I didn't want to hear that damn heart-rate monitor and watch my contractions ebb and flow on a piece of graph paper. My husband and I had done our homework, and we believed that our birth belonged in our home. The only home-birth babies the ER sees are the ones for whom things go terribly wrong. And things go terribly wrong in the hospital, too.

Sunday night, a week past my due date, I watched a movie on

my hands and knees. When I woke up at 1:00 a.m. to pee, the baby had sloshed over to my left side, and I was having mild contractions. Maybe tomorrow will be the day, I thought sleepily, though by this point my hormonal mind had convinced me that I would be the first woman never to go into labour. At 3:00 a.m. the contractions were strong enough to keep me from sleep, but they were still pretty irregular. Later I woke my husband for some company, and we went for a walk around our property. As day broke we listened to the roosters sounding off and watched the bats head home. My contractions went from thirteen minutes apart, to ten, to five. At home, I grabbed my purple ball every time a contraction hit and rocked or bounced through it. Jamin grabbed my hands and squeezed, telling everyone loudly, "My mom is having a contraction!"

The birthing suite, as we now referred to our bedroom, was a busy sanctuary. My husband was making decisions and delegating tasks. Brett, my brother-in-law, was the caterer for this special birthday. We had planned the menu weeks before: tarragon lime chicken salad, sweet potato salad, and lemon chestnut birthday cake. My friend Kathy was there for emotional support and to take pictures. Each of our children had a grandma as a support person, and they could come and go as they pleased.

Marijke and Stacey, her assistant, were absent when I got into the birthing tub. Watery hands massaged me, "taking the edge off," the way I've heard my friends describe an epidural. With my relaxation came a shift, and I began to feel pressure with each contraction, like I wanted to push. I got out of the tub and asked someone to call to find out how far away our midwives were. Kathy and Kurt reached for the emergency home-delivery procedures. The midwives had told me that third babies were "wild cards," so I had no idea what was coming.

"They're in the driveway," my brother-in-law informed me.

I watched out my window as Marijke's white SUV zoomed down our drive. Relief flooded me, and my water broke. Release. I was moaning and growling with contractions now. Each contraction had a different sound; I had never noticed that during previous births. Kurt slid behind me in the tub as I pressed my feet against the opposite side and felt the baby's head moving down.

I told Marijke, "I'm not pushing this time, but the baby seems to be coming down."

She smiled at me, "You don't have to push, your body knows exactly what to do."

There was such freedom in those last minutes. Freedom from counting while pushing, as if it was some regimented exercise, not an organic one. Freedom from the heart-rate monitor ca-chunking through each contraction. Stacey monitored me in the water with a Doppler, and I was barely aware of her presence. Freedom from exams; there was no question that I was fully dilated. Freedom from clocks. I knew by the sun that it was still afternoon, but I had no idea whether I had been pushing for one hour or five. Clearly it didn't matter. None of the numbers mattered.

I threw my head back over Kurt's shoulder, and Marijke encouraged me to reach down and feel the head. I was aware that all I had to do was let it happen. I felt this slimy walnut emerging, and I grinned; it was another first in labour. With the next surge, the head was out, and Marijke suctioned the baby; all clear.

Finally her body slid out in the ultimate release. She swam through the water with Marijke and up onto my chest. Kurt and I cried out in joy. My brother-in-law got so excited he dropped a tray of devilled eggs and rushed in. "Get the kids!" I exclaimed.

Soon the birthing suite was full of activity.

"Wait!" I said, "Does anyone know whether it's a boy or a girl?"

"Who cares?" someone said. "It's a baby!"

While I thought that was rather amiable, I needed proof that this was the daughter I had been dreaming about; it was the female spirit that had been speaking to me since conception. And lifting up her little hips, I saw that she was indeed my Ahna Brie.

I could smell Ahna's birthday cake wafting in, as hands helped me out of the tub and to my couch. There I pushed out the placenta, and Stacey took Ahna to my family. Big sister Maya got to hold her first, as promised, then Jamin, then Grandma. When Ahna was handed back to me, I was ready to nurse her. The kids inspected the placenta with interest. There had been no episiotomy, no hemorrhaging, no blood vessels popping in my eyes. I was able to walk to the bathroom and pee. I felt invincible!

The morning after birth, the sun streamed in through the skylight by my bed; I was the first one awake. I thought about my son chanting, "*Ong namo guru de namo*" (I bow to the divine wisdom inside) to his sister moments after the birth. I pictured my daughter, now a big sister, watching it all in wonder. And then I looked at Ahna tucked between us in bed, and I cried.

I look at my home differently now. As I type this memoir, I am only a few feet from where I delivered Ahna. There is a special energy in that space. I look forward to the time when

Ahna comes home from kindergarten and asks, "Where was I born?" Taking her hand, I will lead her to the space between the pellet stove and the French doors and say, "Right here."

Some people say I am a "brave pioneer woman," while others look askance at the middle-class, educated woman birthing at home: isn't that just for women in communes? This birth was not better than the other two, I remind myself. With Jamin I learned about resilience, and with Maya I learned about patience. This birth taught me that I could trust my body to do everything perfectly.

As an exercise in my third trimester, I had written an account of my perfect birth complete with all the important details. When I reread it later, I realized I had been gifted with a day in which life surpassed art.

Elijah's Birth
by Mollie Dietz

I woke up early on November 30, 2008. My first thought was "I'm still pregnant." Groan. My due date had been November 18, the day before my own birthday. The phone calls from my sister, mother, and mother-in-law had been everyday occurrences during the last two weeks. I had been mentally prepared to give birth since early November, since I knew full-term babies could come as early as thirty-eight weeks. Now I was mentally and physically tired, sore, and uncomfortable.

It was 7:00 a.m. and I needed to pee again. When I wiped, something felt really weird. On the toilet paper was a globby thing with red in it. "Oh, my gosh! I'm glad they warned us what the bloody show would look like," I thought. I told my husband, Chad, that I thought something was finally happening. I called the Greenhouse Birth Center (GBC) and Shelie called me back. I told her about the bloody show and that I was starting to feel mildly crampy. She said that it sure sounded like something was starting, and to keep her posted. That whole day I felt fine except for mild cramps, like I was about to start my period. One thing that surprised me was that the bloody show kept coming the whole day. I finally called Shelie that evening to tell her about it, and she said it was normal. I went to bed that night feeling a strange mix of anticipation, anxiety, excitement and relief that being pregnant was finally coming to an end.

The following morning, Monday, December 1, I woke up at 5:00 a.m. to Chad's alarm. He asked how I felt and if I wanted him to stay home from work. Even though the offer was tempting, I didn't feel any different. I told him to go to work, but to call throughout the day to hear about my progress. He was taking two weeks off, unpaid, after the birth so I knew he needed to get all the hours he could in the meantime.

I fell back asleep, and woke up again around 7:30 a.m., restless. I never had an "energy surge," which some women experience prior to giving birth, but I certainly felt like I needed to be up and walking. When Chad called during his first break at 8:00 a.m., I told him I felt pretty awake and alert. I also thought I could sense a slight pattern starting with the cramps. After we hung up, I called the GBC to let them know what was going on. Kip called me back within a few minutes. She told me to eat and drink plenty and to get back to bed. The last advice I didn't like very much; I wasn't very comfortable when lying down. I lay down anyway and managed to sleep another hour and a half, only waking up during contractions. When Chad called at 10:00 a.m., I knew there was a definite pattern and I couldn't stay in bed any longer. I kind of wanted him to come home, but he asked if I would be okay on my own for another hour and a half until his lunch break.

I had spent the morning walking around the apartment doing little tasks and making sure I had everything in my labour bag. By 10:00 a.m., I had to lean on something, sway and moan during contractions. A couple of times I had a fleeting thought that perhaps the neighbours in our apartment complex could hear me, but by that point I didn't really care. Chad called at 11:30 a.m. and I told him in no uncertain terms to come home now. I wanted him home as I felt we would be leaving for the birth centre in the very near future. I even had a couple of contractions while on the phone.

He was home fifteen minutes later, but I had gone back to bed as an attempt to get a bit more rest. I was in a semi-conscious state between contractions. They were much more intense when lying down, but I needed to rest. I don't remember much starting around the time when Chad came into the bedroom. At some point I asked him to start timing my contractions. He did, and each contraction was longer and more intense than the last. They were not very far apart, maybe four to seven minutes. After a particularly hard one, I asked him how long it was. He replied, "Almost two and a half minutes."

I had had enough. "Call the birth centre, I want to be there now!"

While he packed the food we were going to take I managed to get out of my robe and dress myself. Boy, I sure hated having clothes on by that point! I double-checked my labour-bag list and, certain I had everything, put it next to the door. We left at 2:30 p.m., and at first the ride was okay. That is, until five minutes later when I had my first contraction in the car. I desperately wanted to get out of there!

We arrived at the GBC at 3:00 p.m. I felt like running to the "Green Room," the room I had chosen ahead of time to give birth in. I had a contraction right inside the door and had to lean on the back of the couch in order to deal with it. I couldn't sit very long, but once inside the Green Room I managed to sit long enough for Audra to take my blood pressure. As quickly as I could, I tore off those clothes and got into the long beach cover-up T-shirt I had brought. It was the only shirt that was long enough to afford me some modesty and comfort. I knew I wanted to be in the tub eventually, but I didn't feel a strong urge to get in for about an hour or so.

In the meantime, I walked around and Chad held me in different labour positions during the contractions. I hung from him; sometimes from his neck while facing him, and sometimes he'd hold me under my arms while I'd face away from him. I never knew what I needed until I was in the "wrong" position and had to switch immediately to another. After a while, I was feeling tired again and wanted to sit between contractions. I tried to sit in the rocker but that was not what my body wanted—I hadn't stood up so fast in my whole last month!

Audra brought me the birthing ball and that's just what I needed right then. Pretty soon I felt like I badly wanted to be in that tub. The fifteen minutes it took to fill the tub seemed like forever. I had a sleep bra on under my shirt, so I left my shirt on the floor and got in as fast as I could. Ahhhhh, relief! I loved the feeling of the warm, comforting water and my contractions were not nearly as intense. I could still feel them, but I moaned much more softly.

Chad was so great. He made sure I drank enough water and he held my hand. He helped me out of the tub, to the toilet and back. I hated getting out of the tub. My contractions were so much harder out of the tub that I hurried as fast as I could to pee and then rushed right back in.

At one point, I had a contraction on the toilet. It got more and more and more intense. It was all I could do to hang on to Chad and moan. At the climax I felt a sort of pop and release. It didn't really hurt, but it surprised me. I screamed when it happened. My water broke into the toilet. When I realized what had happened, I thought, "Oh, how convenient." When Chad told Audra, she said not to flush, as she needed to check it to make sure it looked normal. I got back in the tub, not knowing what was going to happen next, but I completely trusted my body and the midwives.

After my water broke, things really got serious. I don't have many clear memories after this point because my brain was soaked with all those wonderful endorphins. I remember looking into Chad's eyes during some really intense contractions. He told me later how hard it was for him to see me go through that. He wanted to cry and take away my pain. It never seemed painful in the way we normally think of pain, though. It wasn't bad. Nothing was wrong. My body was birthing a baby and had to work hard to get him out. All the same, I also saw the love in Chad's eyes; he was with me no matter what and was proud of what I was accomplishing.

Chad noticed I was sweating and asked Audra for some cold cloths. She brought two, and a small bowl of cold water. That was a wonderful feeling. Chad would wipe my face and leave the cloth on my head or over my eyes, always knowing just what I needed. I remember some of my contractions being very close together, about thirty seconds apart, and not being ready for them. Only later did I realize that this was transition.

A short while later I realized that my body had started pushing. I remember having to sit up in the tub with my contractions because my *body* was pushing at that point. I wasn't doing anything on purpose. Chad helped me to sit up, supported me, and helped me to relax back into my semi-reclining position. A few times, during the harder contractions, my eyes sought out one of the midwives. By then Kip, Clarice, and Audra were in the room with me, knitting. Kip was the one in my direct line of sight. She didn't need to say anything although a couple times she gave me an encouraging smile. That's all I needed from her. That was my reassurance that everything was normal, I was going through what countless other women had gone through to birth their babies. Her peacefulness calmed me and helped me in moments of doubt.

I remember Clarice asking if she could check me to make sure the baby wasn't stuck. I was worried when I heard this, worried that her hand would make the contraction worse. I'd previously had no interest in having my dilation checked; however, after the following contraction, I gave her my consent. She checked on the next one and told me the baby was moving down just fine. I remember looking at my belly and noticing that where the bump of baby had been was now flat as the bump had moved down quite a bit. That was so exciting to see!

Kip suggested that I get into a different position as that might help the baby come out sooner. I didn't want to, but on the next contraction my body practically threw itself into that position. I went from semi-reclined to on my knees leaning over the side of the tub. From this position, I was able to cling to Chad as he whispered encouraging words to me. I was also able to look directly at the wall-hanging in the Green Room. It read, "I am not afraid; I was born to do this: Joan of Arc." That gave me new courage and determination during fleeting moments of self-doubt. I could never fully put into words what that meant to me during the hardest part of my labour. It almost brings me to grateful tears just thinking about it.

The active pushing was the hardest work I've ever done. That part was painful and I sometimes got carried away. The midwives had to keep reminding me to take my break between contractions and to push with them. I had fleeting thoughts of, "Just cut the kid out," but then my rational mind would come back and I knew I didn't really want that. I'm sure I made Chad temporarily deaf in his right ear from all the yelling and groaning, but he didn't complain. I had a feeling I was going to be fairly vocal during labour, but while actively pushing I even surprised myself. At one point, I remember yelling, "Get out!" to the baby. Chad told me later that everyone smiled when I yelled that. Most of the time, I yelled for God. It was my way of asking for His help and strength. I also remember thinking, "It really does feel like I'm taking the biggest crap in the world," but that thought did little to console me.

Clarice was the midwife watching for the baby and she encouraged me to reach down and touch as the baby crowned. I never felt his head when it was actually out, but I did feel the bulge when his head was close to being out. Frankly, I wanted to be done with the business of birthing and wanted to hold my baby already!

The pressure kept building and when I couldn't take it anymore, Clarice said, "The head's out! Okay, shoulders next.

You're almost done." I don't remember feeling the "ring of fire," probably because of the water. Though I do remember feeling myself stretch and stretch; I was a little scared that I would tear, but I couldn't stop pushing.

Then, I felt his little body slip, and all of a sudden relief flooded me, the baby was out! I felt his little leg against mine and the umbilical cord brush past me. I scooped him out of the water and sat back. His eyes were wide open, taking in the sudden change of environment. He didn't cry or wail, just looked at us as we looked at him. He protested when Clarice suctioned his mouth, but that was it. I couldn't believe it. My mind couldn't wrap itself around the fact that the work was done and here was my baby. I just stared at him, trying to take it all in. It felt like I was in a dream, waiting to be woken up.

Then I looked at Chad; it was a moment I'll always remember. Even though we'd found out our baby's gender ahead of time, I checked anyway, and sure enough, we had ourselves a little boy: Elijah David. After he was born, it was like a switch had been flipped. I felt calm, happy, hungry, and couldn't stop looking at my son and my husband. It is said that delivering the placenta is the third stage of labour, although it felt more like an afterthought. Chad didn't think he'd want to cut the cord, but he jumped at the opportunity when the midwives asked. Elijah was born at 9:08 p.m. Total labour: thirteen and a half hours.

I hated to get out of that tub, but it had turned really red and the baby needed to be warmed up and dried off. In bed, I shook like I do when I'm very cold, but the midwives said that was normal. The warm sheets felt amazing. After a little while, they had Chad help me to the bathroom, where I fainted on the toilet.

It really scared Chad and I don't really remember being helped back into bed. After about three glasses of juice and some dried apples I started to feel a bit better. Chad watched me until colour came back into my face. I ended up with a second-degree tear and had to be sewn up. That was not fun. Chad held Elijah while Clarice did her thing and I sure wished I could've switched places with him.

After a while, the midwives weighed and measured our baby, but all on the bed. He was 8 pounds, 4 ounces and 20.5 inches long. He was never taken from us; if I didn't have him, then Chad did. Elijah latched right on and nursed for about five minutes. We had the first two hours with him, while my family was busy making my supper of choice: potato soup! We had brought the ingredients and everyone set to work while we waited. Finally, I gave Chad the okay to let everyone in. I felt all right about everyone taking their turn holding Elijah, but I didn't let him out of my sight, and it was a relief when I had him back in my arms.

My best friend, Kacie, was the last to leave at 1:30 a.m. Then, we settled in for the night. It was snowing and the roads were really bad. We snuggled into bed with our hours-old son. Audra was in the next room if we needed anything. It was the perfect start to our baby's life.

The Birth I Wanted
by Caroline Grant

It was dark when I woke up, and for a minute I couldn't figure out what had roused me. My husband, Tony, lay beside me sleeping, and I could hear Ben, our three-year-old, snoring softly in the next room. I waited a beat, listening to the house, listening to my body. Did I need to pee? Had my leg cramped up?

Then before my brain could articulate another question, a wave of cramps and nausea gripped me.

I was in labour.

"Shit," I thought. "I am way too tired for this."

I had been going to my doula Britt's prenatal yoga class every week and feeling pretty limber and stretchy at this point in my pregnancy. She'd taught me how to breathe through my frequent mid-pregnancy ligament pulls, and I'd made a habit of starting the day with a few Cat-Cow Poses to stretch out my sore back. But at the most recent class, I'd felt sick with the flu, and made no promises about coming back.

My due date was still ten days away, but Ben had come so early that waiting for labour was an unfamiliar experience. I had a birth plan in place—friends ready to care for Ben, Britt and her backup's phone numbers programmed into my cell—but I kept wondering when I'd have to set it in motion. A friend of mine thinks constantly about earthquakes, making sure that she has a getaway plan for wherever she is, and I felt a bit like that, although without the worry, just curiosity. At the grocery store, at the nail shop getting my toes painted a soothing seashell pink, driving across the bridge to yoga, I'd wonder, "What would I do if I went into labour now?" Unlike my prepared friend, though, my idle curiosity never moved much beyond, "It sure would be inconvenient to go into labour here!"

Now, I was tired from the full day and cranky at being woken. Yoga abandoned me for a moment when I realized I was in labour. I resisted. I didn't want it to happen right now. I started to bargain with my body a bit. "Please, couldn't I get a little more sleep? You know there isn't going to be much sleep after this baby comes. Please, couldn't you hang on just a little longer?"

Another wave of cramps in reply. I remembered who was in charge of this process. Time to focus on the baby.

My second pregnancy had felt so different from my first: queasier at the start, more comfortable the last few weeks, a much more active baby that we referred to as Thumper. I was certain I was carrying a girl, and Tony and I hadn't yet settled on a boy's name. Josephine, I had considered, or maybe Charlotte. "Come gently to me, baby," I thought to her, and then, "Hey! I've got a birthing mantra!" I was so pleased with myself that I repeated it quietly a few more times. "Come gently to me, baby; come gently…"

Ouch. Baby wasn't listening. I nudged Tony. "I think it's time."

I curled up on my side, fetal position, and Tony came around to kneel by the side of the bed.

"Should we call Britt? How are you feeling?"

"It's too early to call her. Let's let her sleep."

I lay still, holding Tony's hand, not resisting now, but relishing the last few moments before the expected flurry of activity began.

When I'd first suggested to Tony that Britt, my yoga teacher through two pregnancies, be our doula he had felt reluctant and concerned about losing our privacy. "We did fine having Ben, just the two of us," he pointed out. "But it's already more than just the two of us," I reminded him. "There's Ben to think of now. Plus, we're already going into this thing so much more tired than we were delivering him. I want a bit of pampering. I want somebody focused just on me, so that you can think about Ben, or make phone calls, or just sit in bed and stroke my head. She's really a doula for both of us," I suggested. "She can get us snacks, she can run interference with the medical staff. She'll help create and then protect the private space we both want." I wore him down gently, and Britt's calm reassurance about her role finally won him over.

Britt came over several times to discuss the baby's birthday. We'd sit right outside the kitchen, under the redwoods in the shady backyard, talking comfortably while pine needles and the occasional small spider dropped down onto the table. We talked about my labour with Ben, about a quick delivery made unnecessarily quicker by a last-minute episiotomy that I regretted. Despite that, I wasn't ready to consider a home birth; I still wanted the medical support of the hospital in case anything went wrong. I wanted a space away and apart from both Ben and home while I delivered our child. But, because of Ben's speedy arrival, I was concerned about getting to the hospital in time.

Basically, I wanted to sail in, birth the baby with a quick push or two, and then lie back on fresh sheets for a couple days while people fed me and wrapped me in warm blankets. Britt's experience and quiet demeanour made me feel certain that we could both create the peaceful space that I wanted, and resist interventions with which I was uncomfortable.

We talked about timing and logistics, about how often we'd check in with her when the first labour signs began (very often!), about labouring in the big tub at home for a bit before heading to the hospital. Britt made a note to herself to stick her birth kit in the car, just in case; she'd just bought a small SUV, and knew there'd be room to drive us all, me reclining in the back, over the bridge and into the hospital. We talked about how I'd cultured positive for group b strep, and my concerns about needing IV antibiotics if my waters broke early in labour. I didn't want to risk our baby's health, but I knew an IV would both limit my movements during labour, and quite likely expose me to further interventions. Britt suggested dietary changes that might decrease the bacteria level, such as reducing or eliminating sugar and yeast. But, glancing at the rhubarb pie I'd just pulled from the oven, its crust caramelized with cinnamon and sugar, and at the bowl of bread dough rising on the table, she laughed and said, "It might be less stressful for you just to get an IV than to change your cooking and eating habits!"

Time passed as Tony and I lay quietly on the bed together. He rubbed my back and thanked me for picking a more comfortable place than the bathroom floor, where we'd spent the early hours of Ben's labour. I didn't want to call Britt too early, didn't want to wake the friends who would be watching Ben, and didn't want to wake Ben, but I wasn't quite sure of the right time for all the phone calls. Somewhere in my mind I noted what a *mother* I was being, how different already this labour was than my first, when it was just Tony and me. This birth already seemed to involve a crowd of people, a thicket of responsibilities.

I'd dreamt of labouring while in the tub, but my contractions intensified so quickly that I began to worry about getting to the hospital on time. I rode them out, Tony lying next to me and stroking my head until 5:00 a.m., which I decided was an acceptable time to call people and make public this baby-birthing. We called Britt first. Tony spoke to her, then put the receiver where she could listen to me. I'm not sure I actually spoke, but she determined that she had enough time to shower and give her dog, Leo, a quick walk before meeting us at the hospital. Then we called Michael, the friend who'd be watching Ben. Michael and Tony have been friends since they were boys, and he and his wife have a son just ten days older than Ben. It took me as long to shuffle from the ground-floor bedroom to the front door as it took Michael, woken from a sound sleep, to drive the quarter mile to our house. We met at the door and he watched me for a moment helplessly trying to lift my feet into my pale green sandals before crouching down and sliding them onto my feet for me. "Wow," he said quietly, a look of awe mixed with pity on his face, "You're really in this, aren't you?"

Meanwhile, Tony wrote a note for Ben that read: "Dear Ben, Thumper is coming! Daddy is taking Mama to the hospital. They have a big elevator there. We'll come back and get you soon. Have fun playing with your friends. We love you! Mama and Dada." I picked a sprig of jasmine from the vine that climbed up the side of the house and buried my nose in it for the drive into the city.

This was the part I'd been dreading. When Ben was born, we'd made the seven-minute drive to the hospital while I was in transition; I'd put my feet up on the dash and held a washcloth to my face, trying hard to distance myself from my body, the car, everything. Ben was born less than ninety minutes after we got to the hospital. Now I was facing a twenty-five-minute drive, on the freeway and across the Golden Gate Bridge. I was afraid of giving birth in the car with only Tony, and maybe the highway patrol, to help me. I willed Tony to drive quickly, drive smoothly, to distract me with music, to talk about the weather, our coming child, our existing child Ben, and to shut up. I peppered him with impossible and contradictory requests. He kept his hand reassuringly on my knee and drove, keeping up a quiet stream of talk. I had my eyes shut, the window wide open, alternately sniffing my jasmine and leaning out like a puppy to breathe in the cool air. When I realized we were on the bridge, I made myself open my eyes so that later I could tell our baby what kind of day it was. The bridge, lit by the rising sun, glowed deeply orange. The ocean sparkled in the light, all diamonds and sapphires. I felt a wave of joy and happiness surge in me for the day, for the baby, and for our good friends to care for Ben. "We are so lucky, Tony," I said, tears springing to my eyes. "We are lucky, lucky, lucky."

Britt was waiting for us at the Emergency Room entrance, all blond curls and bright pink scarf in the dark concrete space. "You look pretty," I told her, and I wondered if she made that little effort for all her labouring mamas, the way we get pedicures so we have something nice to look at when we're pushing (as if you can push a baby out with your eyes open). She helped us inside, having called ahead, and a nurse greeted us at the door. The stale hospital smell of boiled peas overcame me and I threw up in the hall, all over the floor and onto my pretty green shoes. I wasn't embarrassed at all; in fact, I was rather satisfied, thinking this was a clear sign that I was in transition. I figured I'd have a baby by breakfast. But I could tell the nurse was annoyed with me for not waiting until she'd gotten a basin. I wanted to tell her, "This is how the day will go. I don't normally throw up in public, but as it turns out, today I'm having a baby. My body is in charge. I cannot be polite. I cannot be deferential. You'll just have to keep up." But of course, I couldn't possibly articulate such a fierce sentence; I just waved away the basin she offered too late, and kept moving down the hall to my room as if I owned the place, as if I actually knew where "my room" was. I heard the nurse say something about triage, about checking to see if I was really in labour, and I just gave Britt a pointed look and heard her say politely, "This is her second child. She knows she's in labour." The nurse wasn't pleased, but she gave us a room and Britt immediately went to fill the tub for me.

We kept having little conflicts with the nurse, and Britt kept backing me up. The nurse wanted me on an IV, convinced that because I'd thrown up I was becoming dehydrated. I made a deal with her: if I couldn't keep fluids down, I'd consider it. She brought me a cup with measurements marked on the side so that she could track my fluid intake; later, she stuck a measuring pan in the toilet, too. She wanted to check how dilated I was; I managed to tell her I'd been four centimetres at my recent checkup and to please leave me alone right now. I needed to recover from the drive.

I laboured in the warm tub a long while, the Jacuzzi that had seemed so enormous on our hospital tour now enveloping my labouring body, a tiled cocoon for Tony and me. Once I finally climbed out, my fingers and toes wrinkled like a newborn's, I stood for long stretches, leaning on a big red birthing ball, on Tony, and on the back of a chair. When I found a comfortable spot, I'd stay there for what felt like hours, with Britt and Tony taking turns rubbing the small of my back, my shoulders, and my head. They never took their hands off me, offering support and encouragement with their steady touch. When the contractions grew too insistent, we'd all look together for another position that might help me handle them. My movements were slow, like an underwater dancer; I'd check in with myself after every little shift: does this feel okay? Does this? I'd ease into position, feel it for a moment or two, then adjust if I wasn't yet comfortable. I found myself at one point moving surprisingly into a warrior pose: legs wide, one bent at the knee, both arms outstretched. "Really?" asked Tony, marvelling. "Really," I murmured quietly, eyes closed in concentration. "It seems to be good."

Throughout the day, my contractions would surge for thirty or forty minutes at a time, and then ebb. Britt and I once talked about visual imagery that might help me. "I like the beach, and you're a surfer," I had suggested, "maybe you can talk to me about the ocean?" She never needed to. I felt it right there in my body, waves of contractions building, gripping my body, and then receding. When I felt them subside, I'd lie down to rest, and then, inevitably, the medical staff would descend. They wanted to check my cervix, measure my contractions, tally my fluid intake and output. No longer resisting my body, I resisted what outside interference I could. The nurse would look askance at the numbers from the monitor and say briskly, "Your contractions aren't very strong, are they?"

Britt was always right in my ear, whispering, "The baby is letting you rest, your body is letting you rest, this is a good thing." I'd nibble on the cranberry-nut bar I'd brought, take some more sips of icy cranberry juice and water, then get up and walk off another round of contractions. We'd brought a CD player but, of course, forgot our CDs. Luckily Britt had a couple in her car; Aretha Franklin and Erykah Badu gave me some energy to get through the waves of contractions. I remember leaning on Tony, swaying a slow dance to "Natural Woman."

"This is us," I whispered to Tony, crying happily. "This is us, having our baby." When the waves passed, I'd lie down to recover, even doze off.

The weight of responsibilities I'd felt earlier in the day lifted; I was basking in our little world outside of time. The room had a huge window looking out on the sunny day, and Britt kept spritzing the room with lavender water so it didn't even smell like a hospital. Every once in a while Tony would duck away from the bed to call family and friends with an update. One was in town from Brooklyn, leaving that night. Her son was six months older than Ben, and her second would be three months younger than this child. We'd been through everything together with our first boys, and I sort of wanted to produce a baby for her before she left for the airport. Michael and his wife, caring for Ben, would check in to reassure us about Ben. I could overhear everybody's surprise that my labour was, well, a labour. But, I was enjoying myself. "What a day we're having!" I kept saying to Tony, "What a surprising, amazing day."

Mid-afternoon, one of the residents recommended breaking my waters to move things along, but knowing that this increases the risk of infection, I turned this intervention down. I was starting to feel discouraged, though. Somebody had checked my cervix and I was only six centimetres dilated. I'd been working twelve hours for only two centimetres! I'd done that in my sleep with Ben! Britt and Tony sensed my change in mood and suggested a distraction. We embarked on a long, slow tour of the fifteenth floor of the hospital, peeking in on other labouring women, waiting relatives, new families. My legs felt like sandbags when we returned to the room, and I went straight back to the tub. Britt turned out the lights, Tony sat on the floor holding my hand, and I dozed off for nearly an hour. I didn't realize it at the time, but Britt was right outside on the couch acting as a gatekeeper by fending off the nurses and doctors who wanted access to me. When I finally woke and climbed out of the tub I was bleeding a bit, and then as I leaned over to climb back into bed, a big clot of blood splattered onto the floor. Britt went to tell the attending doctor, and came back to report, "The doctor nearly peed her pants, she was so happy!"

My contractions intensified and I was having a harder time handling them. I started feeling the urge to push, but was told I wasn't yet complete, and so I tried short, focused breaths. This was by far the hardest part—all the yoga in the *world*, I thought, couldn't stop my body from doing what it wanted to do. After a day of giving over to my body and the baby, a day of letting myself be carried along by their waves, I had to focus and resist. The baby was urgent, wanting to twist down and out through the birth canal, 8 pounds of pressure insisting on its right of way. I felt frustrated, stuck, every fibre in me wanting to push the baby out, but also frightened of pushing too soon and tearing myself open.

I knelt against the upright back of the bed, staring into Tony's eyes, clutching his hands, getting strength from him. It was probably only ten minutes, but it felt like hours. I kept begging someone to check, check again, and check again till at last I heard, "You're complete!"

"What does that *mean*?" I wailed. "Can I push? Can I push? I'm pushing!" Britt reminded me that I'd been looking forward to pushing—my favourite part of my first labour—and urged me to enjoy it. It felt great to relax, to open up and bear down.

The doctor said she could feel the baby's hair already. "There's a lot, and it feels curly!" Britt had been at the head of the bed next to Tony, wafting peppermint oil under my nose to give me energy, but now she placed warm compresses on my perineum. She wound up almost catching the baby, he came so fast. His head burst out with an audible pop, a cork from a bottle, breaking the bag of water. The rest of him slithered out as if down a water slide, with just another easy push. The doctor held him up, one hand under his butt, the other supporting his head, to show Tony while someone else helped me turn around, swinging my leg carefully over the thick umbilical cord, so that I could sit down and hold him without cutting his cord.

He was a bit gooey with vernix, with a haze of downy fur on his body and reddish hair on his head. He was clean and wet from the bath of amniotic fluid in which he'd been born. Holding him, I was dimly aware of the doctor and resident rubbing him gently with soft flannel blankets, making sure that he was lively and awake, but somehow it didn't interfere with my holding him, with my being held by Tony, the three of us wrapped in each other's arms like nested dolls.

He was wrinkled and warm and as I held him to my bare chest he began to nurse without even opening his eyes, then slipped off, mouth open, eyes still shut, worn out from his long day. His hand lay open on my chest, a perfect starfish. His brow furrowed in concentration as the resident continued her gentle ministrations, checking his breathing, his heartbeat. Meanwhile, my placenta slipped out and the doctor laid it by my side so we could admire the baby's amazing former home, the veins branching like a tree across its elastic sac. It was a good five minutes before Elijah opened his gray-blue eyes, my exhausted little whelp of a boy, and I could say hello.

Britt stayed a while, making sure that the three of us were comfortable, and that we had enough food. She took a few more pictures, which made me realize suddenly that she'd been snapping the entire time without my noticing, and talked with us about our amazing experience. Then, with a hug and a promise to check on us the next day, she headed home to walk her dog.

The setting sun cast long blue shadows in the room as we lay in bed together. Eli nursed and dozed; Tony and I just gazed quietly at our beautiful new boy. Eventually, a nurse came to bathe Eli, and as Tony watched over his second bath I took advantage of the time to shower. I let the water run hot as it washed the blood off me, feeling strong on my legs despite having stood through most of my labour. I looked down into the tub, hardly recognizing this space as the same spot I'd lain labouring earlier in the day. I looked down at my body, my belly still big but now empty. It was still me here, in the same bathroom, but suddenly everything was transformed. Euphoria surged in me, joy and pride in myself, my baby, my birthing team. And then I climbed out of the shower, ready to rejoin my new family.

Nic's "Speedy Gonzales" Birth
by Dagmar Diesner

I'd been having contractions regularly throughout the last weeks leading up to my baby's birth. I actually told my midwife I could feel that the baby's head was very low for weeks beforehand, and my worst nightmare was to give birth in the street. Even though it was my second baby, she assured me it would not be that fast. How wrong she was!

Nic was born in fifty minutes. These fifty minutes included waking up to look at the time, and wondering why this baby couldn't give me a couple of extra hours sleep. It was 5:20 a.m. on Easter Sunday. After doing a few minutes of deep breathing and rocking on all fours in bed, I decided to get up to prepare the Easter nest for my four-year-old son. My partner, Massimo, woke up asking if it was time, but I assured him that it wasn't, so he put his earplugs back in and went back to sleep.

At one point I went for a pee and saw a bit of blood on the tissue. Worried that something might be wrong, but still not having any major pains, I asked Massimo to call the hospital. We had planned for a home birth, and therefore the panic of when to go to the hospital wasn't relevant to us. We just wanted to talk to a midwife to find out what the bloodstains meant. While Massimo was on the phone attempting to assess my blood flow

31

to the satisfaction of the midwife, I realised the birth of my baby was well under way.

I started organising for the birth by writing simple directions on how to get to our apartment for the community midwives, but was interrupted by my body's restlessness. I managed to get the burning oil and the relaxing music going before I started grunting and moving quickly around the flat. My four-year-old son, Leo, came out of his bedroom with a storybook asking me to read it.

"I can't," I said, and dialed the number of the friend who was to be taking care of Leo during our baby's birth.

I went to stretch my body along the bathroom door musing, "What the hell was I thinking, planning a home birth without any medication? If this is just the beginning of labour, how much more intense can it get?" This all happened while Leo was watching me. Massimo, meanwhile, was still on the phone with the midwife, and was quickly running out of patience.

I was bent over a kid's chair that was next to the bathroom door when finally Massimo arrived. I immediately demanded he press down on my lower back. Just as he touched me, I abruptly got up stating my need to poo. I squatted next to the bathroom tub holding on to the edge. With astonishment, Massimo asked me why I was not pooping into the toilet. "I can't sit on the seat," I said.

And just like that, the baby came! With the bowel movement my body had opened up and I could feel the baby was coming out. I caught his head. My mind was as sharp as a crystal at that moment. I held his head so it wouldn't fall on the bare bathroom floor, and also to avoid a tear. I remembered reading somewhere that tearing is very likely when the birth is very fast. This crossed my mind immediately.

"Quick, put a towel down, I've caught the baby's head," I said. Massimo grabbed a towel from the hook and put it on the floor. The baby was still inside the sac when it landed in Massimo's arms. With the following push, the sac broke and the tender pink placenta came along in one piece. "Quick! A towel," I said. Leo, who was still standing there watching everything, tried to grab a towel from a hook that was too high for him to reach. Massimo and I helped him get it. I wrapped up the newborn with the placenta and went to lie down in bed while we waited for the midwife to arrive.

It was 6:11 a.m. on Easter Sunday and snowing. Leo went to the baby to put his fingers in his mouth and said, "He doesn't have any teeth!" Two minutes later the friend who was to look after Leo entered the house and I pulled back the blanket, proudly showing him our newborn. He went pale and went straight to make breakfast for Leo.

In the meantime, Massimo called the hospital back to tell them the baby had arrived. The midwife asked, "Didn't you just call?"

"Yeah. We just called."

"Well," she said, "you should call the ambulance right away. They're quicker."

The paramedics arrived only five minutes later, and although I was glad to see them, the closed, cozy and happy atmosphere we'd had became rough and mechanic upon their arrival. With their big black boots still on, they walked into the bedroom and kneeled on the bed to cut the umbilical cord. They asked for a plastic bag to put the placenta into—the beautiful pink lump that fed my baby only minutes before.

The midwives arrived shortly after the paramedics, and began examining the baby and me. Because the birth was so quick we hadn't had time to heat up the house, the water, or the towels. The baby suffered a temperature drop, so the midwives decided to take us into the hospital to warm him up. We could have heated the room in a short time as we had additional heating, but I didn't insist too much on staying at home, as I needed some time alone to digest this incredible experience.

Sure enough, once I had arrived at the postpartum ward I started crying, laughing and vomiting; I was in complete shock. I also needed to digest mentally and emotionally what I had just accomplished without much effort.

Leo, on the other hand, was incredibly joyful, and the sanest of us all. This delivery was incredibly bonding for the three of us, and big brother Leo was so proud. He has since told all his friends about his experience, and still talks often about how his brother Nicola came out of my belly, and always does so with a big smile on his face.

I Have to Tell You Something
by Laurel Dykstra

My children were born after the anti-World Trade Organization demonstrations in Seattle and before 9/11. There weren't a lot of queer parents in my community, but I figured since I had more or less learned to be a lesbian from books that there was no reason I couldn't learn to be a mother from books, too.

Queer parenting throws into high relief the issues of economics, privilege, fertility, adoption, and race, as well as the issues that surround who has, who gets, and who keeps kids in our society. Rather than trying to improve my parental fitness in the eyes of adoption agencies or give a whack—pun intended—of dough to a medical lab for something I could get for free from a friend, I decided to go the "known-donor" route. At twenty weeks I went for an ultrasound appointment with Bruce and first uttered what is now a refrain in our family life,

"Oh Bruce isn't my husband, he's my sperm donor."

Ultrasound seemed like a relatively low-key intervention and as an "older mother" at 34, it would relieve some of the constant pressure to detect and abort an "abnormal" or "disabled" fetus. With my shorts pulled down and my shirt hiked up, I lay on the table while an unfriendly technician slid a lubricated ultrasound transducer across my belly. Above, on the screen, she could have been showing an art film of the inside of owl pellets for all I could tell—erratic freeze frames with a bit of spine, some ribs, a skull, fuzzy gray stuff, ribs, a skull.

Without warning Ms. Bedside Manner turned to me and barked, "You seeing your doctor after this?"

"Um, my midwife, yeah."

"I have to tell you something." Endless pause. "There are two of them in there."

That's how I found out I was having twins, twins who would use twice the earth's resources and could *not* be tossed in a backpack while I carried on with my footloose itinerant activism. The joke was on me and my plans. The next day I checked out all the twins books from the public library.

The most woman-centred pregnancy care I could afford was the midwifery practice associated with my insurance provider, and I was lucky to have insurance at all. Unlike a friend of mine whose care included moulding a natural clay bowl for the umbilical cord, deep breathing to recordings of howling wolves, and making art from her placenta; my experience was pretty straight-up utilitarian. Once I was identified—diagnosed really— as carrying twins, the medicalization of my pregnancy was cranked up and I was transferred, unwillingly, to the insurer's physician's practice.

I cranked up my plans, too. According to the library books, twins are born on average between thirty-four to thirty-six gestational weeks, so I assembled my birth team: me, Bruce-the-donor, and Kim and Mary, two strong, spiritual women in tune with my ideas about birth. Mary is a good friend and Kim is a doula who has attended hospital and home births with many of the women in our community. We developed a fairly detailed birth plan and I discussed it with my assigned doctor. Kim, whose own birth experience was incredibly long and difficult, said my doctor had been great at her son's birth. Although even while he listened to everything I said, I could never tell if he was taking it in or just humouring me.

Apparently *my* twins hadn't read the part in the books about coming early. During the last three months of pregnancy complete strangers had been altogether too happy to call out, "Any day now." But, here I was, still pregnant after 40 weeks. I had tried tea, spicy food, nipple stimulation, masturbation, exercise, meditation, bullying. I was huge, it was hot, and I was ready for these babies to come. No tidy little basketball belly for me. I looked like I had a full-size toy chest strapped to my front. During the last week of my pregnancy I folded in half a bed sheet, cut a hole for my head, sewed up the sides and wore it as a tank top. It fit. After carrying them two or three days beyond full term, with no Braxton Hicks contractions and no pre-labour I finally agreed to schedule an induction.

I admire and support home birth. I think it is completely reasonable for a 34-year-old woman to deliver twins at home, but the point of home birth is to be in a comfortable, safe and calm setting. Compared with Guadalupe House where I lived with ten adults, mostly men, the hospital seemed pretty calm and comfortable to me.

Two days before the induction was scheduled, I woke up at 4:00 a.m. for my third trip to the bathroom; my strategy was to keep my eyelids at half-mast and pretend I was still asleep. Back in bed, I lay down, pulled up the plaid flannel sheet, and thought, "Ick, I didn't wipe very well." I got up and went back to the bathroom, leaking on the way. "Hmmm," I thought, "this is not just pee." Feeling weird, I put on some clean underwear, a pad, wrapped my sheet over my shirt and walked down the long hall and up the stairs to Bruce's room.

"Hey Bruce, I think I'm in labour. My water broke."

"Are you having contractions?" He asked.

"Yeah. But I don't think we need to call anybody yet, we can just hang out downstairs for a while."

"How far apart are they?"

"I'll time them."

"Oh. That was about five minutes. That too. Maybe we should call Mary and Kim then." Bruce climbed down from his loft. Mary said she would shower and meet us. Kim came to the house and we drove the three blocks to the hospital in a whitish car, or maybe gray. I remember it as Mary's car, but Mary wasn't there yet. My memory is not a continuous stream from this point, but bits and pieces, ragged and out of order.

At the night entrance a security guard said something stupid like, "It's that time is it?" It was 5:00 a.m., I was hugely pregnant, wearing a bedsheet and being supported on either side. What the fuck time did he think it was?

Someone put me in a wheelchair. In the elevator I began to feel nauseous and when we got upstairs I called for something to be sick in. They wanted me to fill in some forms, so I puked in my shirt. They took my shirt away and I was bereft with only my sheet.

The first doctor on duty kept trying to attach monitors

everywhere. We resisted by waiting him out. My doctor said later if I had delivered on that guy's shift I would have had a Cesarean for sure. At some point I was moved with my entourage to another room; I was not so impressed. It was a bigger room with more space for machines and people if something "went wrong." I spent a lot of time being unimpressed while in labour, feeling like everyone else had really dumb priorities and requests that were distracting me from the job at hand. I had chosen a powerful painting of a woman as my visual focus point. Instead I fixated on the loops of medical tubing at the head of the bed. I also brought some fancy vitamin-fortified popsicles that I never used. I had planned to have no medication, but boy, after several hours I was sure thinking about it. I made a joke at one point so it couldn't have been that bad.

There are some great pictures of my "team" working with me, and the doctor standing out of the way letting us do it, just like we had agreed. A couple of times he came forward and made a suggestion then backed off again. Because I was so heavy I could not support my weight in a wide deep squat, so he suggested I lie down with my knees up.

Just before the baby was born everyone was cheering, "We can see the head; here, put your hand here so you can feel the head." Someone took my hand and put it there, but I couldn't tell what was what, it was all swollen flesh, blood, and hair. I couldn't tell what was baby and what was me and frankly, I didn't care, I didn't want to touch the baby; I wanted to push it out! Finally with some screaming and some poop and some tearing, I did. Myriam was born.

I had asked not to know the ultrasound technician's

assessment of my children's presenting sex or genitals. I figured there was no point in subjecting my children to gender expectations before birth, as they would start soon enough. As I tell my kids, you cannot tell if someone is a boy or a girl by looking at them, you have to believe what that person tells you. Nevertheless, I had been sure my babies were boys, perhaps because I could not imagine, as a queer feminist, what I would do with twin boys. When they told me the baby was a girl I thought, "Okay, I must be having a girl and a boy."

Basically, I had two very different birth experiences. With Myriam, it was supported, natural childbirth, without medication or intervention and she was born six and a half hours after I went into labour: lusty and loud and ready to nurse.

So the next kid, who for three months had been lined up behind older sister Myriam, head pointed at the exit, ready to go, suddenly found the crowded little room empty and turned around and swam upstream. We tried waiting, massage, and changing my position, but no amount of encouragement or prodding could convince this baby to turn around. Finally, as I had negotiated with the doctor, we decided to attempt a breech delivery. I nursed Myriam, and curled up on my side for an epidural. Lots of people came in for this. After they put in the needle, it took a long time to work; they kept wiping my leg with alcohol swabs and asking if I could feel it. My legs were like huge lumps of bread dough, but with me pushing and the doctor pulling, Harriet was born: feet first and indignant, 45 minutes after her sister.

They held up this red baby—her hair was all standing on end and she was all outraged and hilarious. I said, "Well, that's Harriet."

It was pretty amazing to have had such a low-intervention delivery in a medical setting and to have a twin born breech at age thirty-four, but it was not through any advocacy or virtue of my own. My experience relied very much on the goodwill of the physician to whom I had been assigned. After what felt like a difficult, but kind of triumphant, birth experience, it all became a little bleak.

I was totally unprepared for the placenta. Having given birth to two infants weighing a total of 15 pounds, I was somewhat appalled to have to deliver this other thing. It took a long time and a lot of painful contractions for my huge uterus to return to a normal-ish size. I lay there pitifully, thinking, "But, I already had two babies, I should be finished."

Later some staff person came to me and said, "We need to get this room ready for the next person. Do you think you can sit up?"

Ever accommodating I answered, "I think so." When I tried I nearly fell off the bed, I had lost so much blood.

They took me downstairs at about noon. Mary and Kim had gone to work. Bruce went home to sleep and I felt like, "Hey don't leave, I just had two babies, the show is not over, I just accomplished a really hard job and nobody is staying to help me." People came to see me and the babies as though all the work was done and the products were available for viewing, but I don't remember much of that day. At some point I had a blood transfusion.

Suddenly it was night.

I had read a great deal about twins regarding labour and

delivery, but nothing about newborns or what to do with them. My friend Tara came and spent the night at the hospital, but I still felt like I was alone in the dark and outnumbered by two tiny creatures with floppy limbs and silly hats who wouldn't stop crying and wouldn't tell me why.

Far-From-Home Birth
by Ginny Kaczmarek

When my water broke the morning of September 2, 2005, I was five hundred miles from home, and unsure whether I even had a home anymore. Five days earlier, my husband, Ian, and I had boarded up our windows, packed up our cat, family photographs, and a few extra pairs of underwear, heaved my nine-month-pregnant belly into the front seat, and left New Orleans. A storm was coming, and although we hadn't wanted to travel mere days before my due date, the size and ferocity of Hurricane Katrina convinced us that we'd be safer if we left. We assumed we'd return in a few days, before the baby was born, unaware of just how long and difficult our journey would become.

By late night Sunday, August 28, when we arrived at the home of our friends, Aimée and Scottie, in Birmingham, Alabama, Hurricane Katrina had become a Category 5 storm in the Gulf of Mexico, aiming directly for New Orleans. All day that Monday and Tuesday the four of us huddled around the TV, changing channels from one newscast to the next as if someone, somewhere might finally admit that the images we were seeing were a hoax. The levees had broken; the resulting floods were swallowing the majority of our city. Our local Rite Aid Pharmacy was underwater, our nearby Walmart had been torn apart by desperate people. What about our house, we wondered. Was it filled with water? Had someone kicked in the door seeking food, cash, or shelter? As I sat rubbing my belly and staring out the window at the calm, blue Alabama sky, I understood that we weren't going home anytime soon. We needed to find a place to have our baby, fast.

Ian and I forced ourselves to stop watching the horrors unfold on TV and to focus on our most immediate concern. With the baby due in two days, our options for natural childbirth, my preference, were few. Back in New Orleans, we'd planned to have a medication-free water birth in a hospital with a midwife and a doula in attendance. Alabama, however, was a notoriously hostile climate for midwifery. Most of the OBs and maternity nurses we contacted were unsupportive and unwilling to honour requests for intervention-free delivery, citing rigid, archaic hospital policies, such as mandatory internal fetal monitoring, IV tethers, and a catheter. Everyone tried to reassure us that a healthy baby and a healthy mother were all that mattered, but to me, having a healthy birth experience was also important. I didn't want this most personal of decisions to also be swept aside in Hurricane Katrina's aftermath.

After much research, Ian found a team of midwives based north of Birmingham, and we agreed to meet with them the following day. In soft Alabama drawls, Susan and Tanya described their training, their years of experience, and the hundreds of healthy babies delivered. They treated me not as a victim with limited options, but as a woman capable of making choices. Even the baby in my belly seemed to respond positively to the sound of their voices, wiggling softly under my hands.

Because they are lay midwives, not nurse-midwives, Alabama law forbids them from delivering babies in hospitals. Instead, their clients give birth in a small house in Tennessee, another hour away, where lay midwifery is legal. I hadn't originally planned for a home birth, but with the status of our own house in question, spending this most stressful and intimate time in a house with caring, responsible attendants sounded ideal. Excitedly, we came up with a plan for labour and delivery. "Bless your hearts," Susan told us and gave us a key to the house where babies are born.

The morning after we met the midwives, on my official due date, my water broke. Apparently my son had been waiting for just the right moment to arrive.

"What does this mean?" Ian kept asking. "Are you okay?"

I felt fine. No cramps yet. I was giddy and nervous. Part of a Jane's Addiction song popped into my head and wouldn't leave: Perry Farrell shouting, "Here we *go!*" We called our new midwives, who told us to meet them at the Birmingham home of one of their colleagues for a quick exam.

Once we had arrived at the house, Susan took my blood pressure and felt my belly, then listened to the baby with a handheld monitor. Everything looked great, she said, and I still felt fine. Susan told us, "Call me when you get to the house, and let me know when you're ready for us." Despite the popular notions of childbirth as a crisis, it was wonderful to feel as though it wasn't, even if our plan for a leisurely, but long, drive to Tennessee made our friends a little nervous. Because other members of our midwifery team lived along the drive and near the birth house, we knew there'd be help along the way, if we needed any. Ian and I loaded the car, hugged Aimée and Scottie goodbye, and said, "Next time we see you, we will be three!"

Driving through the green hills of Alabama, the sun shining warmly, I felt calm, excited, and hungry. We called our parents and friends, warning them that we didn't want to talk about anything New Orleans related because we needed all of our concentration for the event ahead. For the most part, everyone understood, though it was hard for them to hide their fear for our predicament: giving birth in a strange place among strangers, but not in a hospital. For myself, I was glad to focus on something positive instead of the ongoing catastrophe that our hometown had become.

When we reached Tanya's homeopathic shop, where we'd first met our midwives only the day before, she made sure we had all the important phone numbers, then sent us across the street for lunch. I had started to feel a little crampy, which delighted me— this was really happening! The cafe's owner made the most amazing chocolate milkshake, satisfying my late-pregnancy cravings. When she asked my due date, we laughed and told her, "Today! We're driving to the birth house now." She refused to let us pay for our drinks as our baby's first birthday gift.

We arrived at the birth house in the early afternoon. It was arranged with several rocking chairs, big comfortable beds, a massive whirlpool tub, and lots of books on childbirth and infant care. Most hilarious, and slightly unsettling, was the note by the front door reminding mothers, "Don't forget to take your placenta with you!" After making sure I'd be okay on my own, Ian drove to Walmart and the video store to gather supplies for the next few days. I tried to get comfortable in the house, arranging our supplies, putting away snacks, reading some of the labour books, doing a few of my labour yoga moves. When Ian came back, we began watching Will Ferrell's *Elf*, but about halfway through the movie, my contractions intensified. I stood at the counter dividing the kitchen from the living room and leaned on my elbows, resting my head on the counter and stretching out my back. Ian tried to time the contractions, but neither one of us felt confident that we were doing it correctly, so we gave up. They were definitely coming hard and fast, so we decided it was time to call the midwives.

At about 6:00 p.m., four midwives came to the house, including Susan and Tanya, but stayed out of our way, letting us remain focused on the ritual we'd established. When I felt a contraction starting to build, I would lean on the counter and Ian would rub my back in a very specific pattern as the contraction worked its way through me, drawing on techniques we'd learned in our Bradley birthing classes. If he altered the massage pattern or we didn't get into the position soon enough, the pain was more chaotic and intense. The rest of the world dropped away as we focused on our routine.

Knowing I was interested in water birth, the midwives prepared the whirlpool tub. A quick exam determined that I was dilated to around five centimetres, ready to enter the water. Ian put on a CD, and the music and water soothed me instantly. Ian got in behind me and continued rubbing my back. Not long afterward, I began to feel the urge to push and someone brought out a little birthing stool to put in the tub. Trying not to disturb us, the midwives spoke quietly a few feet away from us, but the whispering made me paranoid. "What is it?" I said, and they told us we needed to get out of the tub. Residual detergent in our clothes (I wore a top and Ian had kept on his underwear) was clouding up the water, making it frothy and soapy. Not good for me or the baby.

They dried me off, all the while trying to maintain our massage rhythm. I moved to the large bed, sitting with my knees up, with Ian behind me. I was fully dilated; the midwives could see and feel the baby's head. It was close to midnight. Someone brought out a camera and took a picture of Ian and me on that bed, sure that the baby would arrive soon. That photo still makes me sad; none of us knew what a long way we still had to go.

After pushing for a while, the urge diminished, and I lay on my side to rest while the midwives conferred. They'd determined that the baby was posterior, facing my front instead of my back, which explained why I needed Ian to massage me; I was experiencing the dreaded "back labour." Because the baby was turned around, the midwives recommended that I push lying back with my knees up, rather than leaning forward, which opposed all of my research. It was very difficult for me to let go, to trust that they knew best. They also said that I had a stubborn cervical lip that wasn't moving out of the baby's way. The next few times I felt the urge to push, Tanya tried to hold the lip out of the way, which was extremely uncomfortable. At the same time, her presence gave me something to focus on, instead of feeling like I didn't know where or how to push. I began to think that my baby was stuck.

During the next several hours, we put those midwives through their paces. Every twenty minutes or so, I'd feel the urge to push and we'd try a new position. I leaned over the back of the toilet, stood in the shower with warm water spraying on my belly, laid on the bed or on the floor. Two midwives held my arms as we stomped through the house to shake my baby loose. We marched up and down the short steps that led to the backyard, walking around the chilly patio. Someone reminded me that I wasn't wearing any pants, but I didn't care. I wasn't being terribly quiet, either, lowing deep throaty moans like a moose in heat. Laura tried a technique that she had learned from Mexican midwives, where she laid me on a blanket, grabbed the sides of it so I was in a sling, then jostled me back and forth in an attempt to get the baby to turn around. It didn't work, but it did make me laugh, not an easy feat given the situation.

Between contractions, I poured out my worries and fears to Susan: how scared we were about our house, how indebted we were to our friends, how guilty I felt about pushing my family away when they wanted to help. I wanted to purge my mind and body of any negativity, in case holding in my feelings was holding in my baby. Still, my labour seemed interminable as wave after wave of contractions exhausted my body and my mind.

Ian was with me every step, massaging my back until (and after) his arms were sore. He uncomplainingly carried out all of my whims, fetching me sips of water, Gatorade, or crackers, turning on the music, turning off the music, warming the shower, turning it off because it was too warm. When I didn't know what I wanted or what to ask for, he patiently was there, staying close to me or moving away a bit if I needed some space. He was my one constant in this bizarre journey, and he was my family, my home, my strength, just as he had promised he would be many years before.

By about four in the morning, however, each new impulse to

push brought with it a feeling of despair. "Oh God, I can't do this," I'd moan, and everyone would whisper, "Yes, you can, you can do this." Sometimes the midwives would instruct me not to push in an attempt to store up my energy. Though we could still feel the baby's head, he wasn't making much progress. When I wanted to curl up and sleep after a particularly gruelling pushing session, Susan and Tanya sat next to me and said, "Ginny, we're starting to see meconium. That could mean the baby is in distress, but not necessarily. His heartbeat still sounds strong and steady. But you might want to decide whether you want to keep on going as you are, or move to a hospital. At the hospital, they might have tools to help you deliver. It's your choice." They did not seem terribly worried, but I was so tired and didn't want to risk my baby's health. Ian and I decided to go to the hospital.

After a harrowing drive, with Ian driving our Volvo and Susan and I trying not to have that baby in the backseat, we arrived. The hospital was so bright that I could barely open my eyes. They squeezed me into a wheelchair while Ian and Susan sorted out the details with the nurses. A male orderly wheeled me to the elevator. People in the lobby were watching me, and I realized that I was fulfilling expectations from TV or the movies: a pregnant woman moaning and puffing as she's wheeled quickly to the maternity ward.

Disappointment washed over me. I had been so excited by the prospect of a home birth, but now here we were, in the hospital. I was touched that all four midwives came with me, even though I was "giving up" on the home-away-from-home birth we had envisioned. But because we had crossed back into Alabama, state law mandated that they could act only as doulas, offering support and comfort, but no medical advice. Losing their counsel unmoored me and, for the first time since my water broke, I felt afraid.

After some disagreements with the nurses about whether I needed a paper gown and an IV pole, I waited for the doctor to examine me. She said that the cervical lip was gone, the baby seemed fine, and I could deliver this baby vaginally in the next couple of hours. The midwives were pleased with the doctor's consideration of my birth plan, but another couple of hours sounded like eternity to me. I was exhausted. I kept throwing up what I thought was red Gatorade but ended up being blood. Nobody seemed particularly worried, except Ian. I whispered to him, "Just cut the baby out of me. I don't want to do this anymore. Just get him out of me." He stroked my hair and hid his wet eyes from me.

The doctor suggested Pitocin to get my contractions moving faster. I hadn't wanted any medication, but I also wanted to be done. I looked to Susan and Tanya for their opinion, but they were frustratingly unable to give me one. Ian said it was up to me. I agreed to a little bit in my IV, hoping it would help. The midwives kept coaxing me into a leaning-back position as we tried different postures in the hospital bed. As I lay back, knees spread, the nurses clucked their tongues at the sight of my swollen, overworked perineum, saying, "Oh honey, you are going to be *sore*."

When the Pitocin kicked in, the contractions came rapidly, relentlessly. I was whizzing down a hill, out of control. I couldn't keep up with the chaotic rhythm anymore. I was pushing without rest breaks, sweating, and throwing up more blood. Someone said, "Look, the sun is coming up," which made me miserable. A mean nurse yelled at me to "Get mad! Get angry! Don't cry! Don't be such a baby!" She seemed to think our gentle approach wasn't working, so she was extra obnoxious to show us how it was done. She roughly yanked open my legs. My midwives were horrified, but helpless. I wanted to kick her. I shouted, "Shut up!"

Suddenly, there was a change. The overhead lights flared on, and the room burst into activity, metallic instruments clanking. I heard, "Get the doctor." I had begun to bleed heavily, and they were worried that the placenta had torn, putting my baby in danger. The doctor arrived, saying, "Okay, let's get this baby out." A huge, white, laser-looking thing emerged from the ceiling. The doctor explained that she was going to use a vacuum to help pull out the baby. Ian, who had been stationed by my shoulder, was suddenly missing.

"Where's Ian?" I asked Laura, and she assured me that he'd be right back. He had become dizzy when he heard that I was bleeding, thinking of my mom who had almost died from hemorrhaging while giving birth to me. My midwives got him some food and drink, and he returned to my side.

Inserting that vacuum meant pulling open my poor perineum, causing a sharp, shooting fire between my legs. I bellowed. That nasty nurse was shouting at me, but my midwives and Ian were all around me, telling me to push, push, push. I put my feet on the flat paddle-like stirrups and curled into a sitting position with each push. Susan told me to force my voice down into my cervix, and I thought I might explode. After what seemed like hours, I felt a burning, splitting-open pulling sensation and a pop, then some rustling between my legs. A baby's shrill cry filled the room.

I said, "Is that him? Is he here?" Everyone laughed and cried as the doctor pulled him out. While the nurses suctioned, wiped, and wrapped him, I leaned forward over my belly, reaching my arms, saying, "Give him to me! Give him to me!" Finally, they did.

I unwrapped him. My eyes had become so accustomed to being squeezed shut, I couldn't focus. He was red and screaming to high heaven, but he was here, in my arms, at last. I lifted my shirt so his skin was next to mine, but he wasn't interested in nursing. Ian reached toward him tentatively, eyes brimming, still stroking my hair. Our midwives snapped pictures of the three of us. Between my tears, I whispered, "Shh, shh, it's okay, it's Mama. Mama's got you." He had all his parts, fingers and toes, pink and wrinkled. I breathed him in and felt like I would never let him go.

The doctor waited patiently for me to deliver the placenta, again impressing my midwives with her willingness to let my body take its time. I thought the placenta would just "whoosh" out, but the contractions proved almost as unpleasant as pushing out the baby. Once it was out, the doctor said that the placenta hadn't torn and the baby hadn't breathed in or swallowed any meconium. He and I were just fine. The midwives guessed that he was at least 10 pounds, so we were all surprised (and a bit disappointed, after almost ten hours of pushing) that he weighed only 8 pounds, 13 ounces. Still, not a small baby! The nurses marvelled at his head size (15 inches), which made me feel slightly more vindicated for my trouble.

After everyone had finally gone, Ian and I were able to turn the lights down low and lean back in the bed, just us, our new family. It was Labour Day weekend, appropriately enough, so the ward was quiet. A kind nurse came in after her shift to help us with breastfeeding; she was a La Leche League leader who had worked with our midwives before. Food came, but they didn't know that I was a vegetarian; I had never had a chance to mention it. Ian and I tried to be friendly and accommodating, but it was a frustratingly delicate balance. Finally, we received the paperwork that allowed us to take our new baby out of the hospital, if not exactly home.

As we were climbing into our car, a man rushed toward us. He and his family, awaiting their own newest addition, had heard about the New Orleanians with a newborn. He pressed a small wad of cash into Ian's hand. "For your baby," he said. He had collected cash from his family members in the lobby on our behalf. We didn't want to take his money, yet we weren't sure how to refuse such kindness and generosity. After thanking him, we drove back to the birth house in silence, confused by our new roles as parents, as refugees.

For a week, the three of us revelled in our "babymoon," almost entirely uninterrupted by external reality. We didn't turn on the TV and asked family and friends to honour our decision to keep the outside world outside. Nonetheless, when I slept, I dreamt of my baby sinking under rough water, floating away from me as I groped for him, my fingers barely brushing his blue lips. I'd wake to find myself awash in sweat and breast milk, my tiny son sleeping by my side. Our freedom from our troubles was limited; we'd soon need to reenter the real world.

On September 9, Aimée's birthday, we drove back to Birmingham with little Emery howling in his new car seat. When we arrived, Aimée and Scottie led us into what had been their home office the week before. White lace curtains billowed over a white crib; dressers overflowed with baby powder, diapers, wipes, and washed and folded baby clothes. While we were gone, Aimée and Scottie had rallied friends, family, and co-workers to donate everything we could possibly need for the foreseeable future. I sat on the edge of the bed, my son in my arms. Aimée put an arm around me and said, "Stay as long as you need to. This house always seemed too big anyway," and I burst into tears.

We stayed with our friends for three months. Days blurred together in a haze of sleeplessness and spit-up, with intermittent reports about the stagnant pond that New Orleans had become. Emery grew from newborn to chubby-cheeked infant by the time New Orleans was reopened to residents. Ian ventured back in October and November to oversee the replacement of our damaged roof and the repair of our waterlogged ceilings. Despite the hassle, we knew that we had gotten off easy. As part of the "sliver by the river," the highest edge of our bowl-shaped city, our neighbourhood had suffered no flooding. Our front door had not been kicked in by looters; rescue teams had not spray-painted a red X across our windows to indicate the number of dead inside. We were grateful, but also felt guilty: Most of the people in the city had lost everything, and we had come through relatively unscathed.

In mid-December, we were finally able to bring our baby home. As we strolled the streets, bought groceries at one of the few functioning supermarkets or grabbed lunch at a reopened po-boy shop, recently returned neighbours would pause to squeeze our baby's plump thighs and tickle his chin to score a precious toothless grin. For a moment, in the midst of so much loss, stress, and pain, we all had something ordinary and miraculous to talk about: teething, sleeping through the night, nursing. The elements of a new life were blossoming. Never before had I felt such a connection to the place I lived, to the people around me. New Orleans had become more than just a place to live; it was a community of survivors. Ian and I decided to demonstrate our faith in our city's resilient spirit by raising our Alabama-born baby in New Orleans. And if we are ever blessed with another child, we hope to welcome him or her to the world in our home, now that we understand that there truly is no other place like it.

Naturally
by Carole Monnier Clark

Lili was born on the lunar eclipse by Cesarean section. This was not a choice, but rather a strong recommendation by doctors because she was breech. She'd been sitting in my belly, pushing her head against my ribs for more than six weeks, with no sign of budging even though I'd desperately tried everything to persuade her that she should turn over. When the ultrasound technician casually mentioned that her bum was where her head should be during my seventh month of pregnancy, I had a sinking feeling that I couldn't shake for the rest of the day. Up until this point, my pregnancy had been going smoothly. Lili had been head down since the fifth month, and I had visions of my natural birth that was going to be as easy and as uncomplicated as my mother's birthing experiences had been.

"Breech baby means a Cesarean," kept repeating in my head, and this thought was truly frightening to me. Everyone around me kept assuring me that she had plenty of time to turn around before delivery, and that things would be fine. I didn't feel fine. I felt like I had to be proactive and get this baby head down, if only to appease my growing anxiety about the complete loss of control over my birth experience that I felt a C-section would be. For weeks leading up to Lili's birth, I underwent as many alternative treatments as my close friend and doula, Stephanie, and I could find. This included homeopathy, chiropractic work, and long hours crawling around on my knees—occasionally in other people's homes during dinner parties when the sitting had been going on just a little bit too long. My very patient husband, Jesse, even agreed to spend twenty minutes every evening holding a glowing hot stick of charcoal only millimetres from my baby toes as prescribed by my acupuncturist, who also gave me the traditional needle treatments.

My entourage was very positive, but as the days passed and Lili's due date approached, my hope for a natural birth was growing smaller and smaller. By this time, my doctor had made it clear that an elective C-section was required to minimize the risks associated with my situation. I'd never heard of making an appointment to have a baby and the very idea of it made me sick to my stomach. I couldn't imagine anything less natural, or opposed to what I had planned for us. Jesse and I discussed our situation constantly, and we both felt that an elective C-section was not for us, even if we were being made to feel that we would be taking unnecessary risks if we waited for labour to begin before having the procedure. Somehow, we managed to convince my doctor to schedule the operation on our baby's due date, February 29, which was a full two weeks past normal protocol. During this time, my emotions were running high and the stress that I was experiencing was having a negative impact on my state of mind and general well-being. Seeing my distress, my acupuncturist suggested that I contact a Birth Intuitive. She described her own birth experience, and told me that speaking to a medium during her difficulties had really helped. I was willing to give it a shot, as I was grasping for any source of comfort.

This phone conversation happened on February 18. We spoke for more than an hour about everything from my energy chakras to my baby's spirit and the reasons for choosing us as parents. The experience left me feeling connected and calm about our circumstances. The one thing that really stuck with me from the entire conversation was when she told me that Lili wanted me to have more fun, like I was having earlier in the pregnancy. She felt that I had become stressed and rigid. She wanted me to move and dance and feel happy again.

That evening, Jesse and I decided to go swimming at the local YMCA to indulge our little daughter and spent hours rolling around and doing flips in the water to show her what to do! As we walked home up the huge hill back to our apartment I felt invigorated, but by the time we reached the top I asked Jesse to run ahead and come back for me with the car, because suddenly I couldn't take another step.

Through the night, I kept waking up to cramps in my lower abdomen that felt a lot like menstrual cramps. When I woke up in the morning, I felt different for some inexplicable reason, and somewhere deep inside I started realizing that this was going to be *the day*. I sat on the couch for most of the day, staring out the window at the frigid minus 20°C weather, and noticing that the cramps I had been feeling the night before kept coming and coming, until finally I started writing down the time after each sensation. Around three in the afternoon, it was clear that these cramps were coming every fifteen to twenty minutes. I called Jesse and told him that I was maybe going into labour. He laughed and said he didn't think so, as it was too early. By the time he got home from work, the cramps were coming every eight minutes. He drew me a bath and reminded me that if we went to the hospital, we would just find ourselves back in the same situation we had been in the previous week, when we had gone to the hospital due to an amniotic-fluid scare and narrowly avoided a C-section right then and there. So, a week later when I told Jesse that I thought my labour was progressing and I wanted to go to the hospital, he wanted me to be really, really, really sure it was actually happening.

I finally put down my fork, looked into his eyes and said, "I know this baby is coming tonight, and I want to go to the hospital right now." The bag was still in the car from the previous week's scare, so all we had to do was hop, or rather lower slowly, into the car and call our doula on the way. Once we arrived at the hospital we were happy to find that the ward was quiet with barely anyone around. We were greeted and settled into a private room where a nurse attached a monitor to me and the intern came in to introduce herself. I explained my situation, that my baby was breech and that I was nine days ahead of my due date, but that I had been feeling contractions since the previous night. The monitor didn't seem to be registering any contractions, even though I felt them with growing intensity, so nobody seemed to be paying much attention to me.

After some time had passed, a nurse checked my monitor and realized that it was sitting on baby's head and therefore not registering contractions because of her breech position. She readjusted the sensor and much to everyone's surprise, other than my own, I was having quite strong contractions. I felt redeemed for the pain that I had been "imagining" up until now, as it was confirmed that I was in labour and two centimetres dilated. Suddenly an ultrasound technician, nurses and the resident doctor crowded our small room. An ultrasound confirmed that she was still bum down, and the option of trying to turn her while administering an epidural was eliminated as her heart rate was showing signs of distress through each contraction. The doctor on call came in at this point and told us very seriously that the time had come and that he was booking us into the operating room during the next slot at 2:00 a.m.

Everything that happened next felt dreamlike and adrenalin-fueled. I was downright terrified as they wheeled me into the OR while explaining the procedures to me. Everything felt cold, infused in fluorescent light and way out of my control. A nurse had me sit on the edge of the operating table rounding my back as the anesthesiologist found a good location to give me the spinal injection. I kept my eyes focused on nurse's pendant, a small red rose on a pink background, trying hard to keep my breath steady and calm while fingers prodded my spinal column and finally inserted the needle. This was the only physically painful moment of the procedure, and it was over quickly as they guided my body into a horizontal position and strapped my arms and legs to the table.

Soon after, Jesse came into the operating room and sat beside me in his scrubs looking just as scared as I was. I started shaking all over uncontrollably, which wouldn't stop until several hours later, a side effect of my fear and the drugs they were giving me to numb my body. For a moment leading up to procedure, I was thinking that the morphine hadn't taken and that I would feel the impending incision. Of course it had and the Cesarean happened within a few minutes. I could feel the tugging and pushing as they opened me up and pulled Lili from my belly. We heard her first cry from the other side of the curtain, and immediately both of us started to cry, too. The doctor came around to show her to me, but had to quickly move her to a station nearby as they were afraid that she had inhaled some meconium. Jesse went with Lili, and I was wheeled off into the recovery room.

This is all a little blurry, but I remember lying there not being able to feel anything past my throat while a nurse aloofly worked on a computer nearby and came to put ice on my forehead and chest every once in a while to see if my feeling was coming back. After an indefinite period of time, I was wheeled down the hall where Jesse met me just as a baby's screaming came into earshot. "That's our daughter!" he said.

We went into the Special Care Nursery where I was shown Lili once again, but I didn't hold her as I hadn't fully regained the use of my limbs. The following hours were spent fitfully shaking in a bed in the postpartum ward. I remember a nurse coming and asking if my face was itchy. It was, I said, I felt like a strung-out addict and she gave me something for it through my IV.

Seven hours after she had been delivered, they brought Lili to me and put her in my arms. It felt so strange to hold this little creature that was mine after all the incongruous events of the night, but regardless, she curled right up against me and started to search for my breast. She latched on as soon as I offered it to her, and I was overwhelmed with relief and joy. Finally, after all the events of the night a moment that felt natural.

Manuel's Birth Story
by Karine Gautschi

It all started at 6:00 p.m., just before my husband, Simon, came home from work. I hadn't had any contractions yet, but I just knew that there was something going on, even though this was my first experience with delivering a baby.

"Women are built to give birth. It is hard work but I will do it. I must trust my body and believe in myself." This mantra had been all I could think of during the last few weeks. I was surprised by the unmistakable message my body sent to me to let me know that I had just entered the birthing process. I felt very connected to my body and regarded this connection as a confirmation of my mantra. It gave me strength.

Simon and I went for a "last" cup of coffee that night at a coffee shop just a few blocks away from where we lived. We knew that our old lives were coming to an end, and we enjoyed the walk and being "alone" for the last time. Later that night, shortly after midnight, I woke up with my first contraction. I got up and left the bedroom so that Simon could sleep, as there was not much for him to do just yet. My contractions lasted about forty seconds and were coming every fifteen minutes which kept me awake all night, and most of the following day. I was amazed at how I was dealing with it all. I kept reminding myself that with each contraction I was one step closer to meeting our baby and that kept me going. Simon was always close by, but I wanted to be alone in order to concentrate on my body. I felt confident—maybe for the first time in my life!

After twenty hours of contractions, we called the hospital to ask how long this could go on because the pattern wasn't changing at all, and there were no other symptoms that would have suggested that labour was progressing. We were starting to run out of patience. We wanted to hold our little guy so badly and at the same time we were a bit afraid of what was coming. We were excited, happy, scared, and restless all at the same time. Our love for one another was stronger than ever. It was just about the baby and us; nothing else mattered. We stayed at home waiting for a new sign of progress that finally came in the form of some vaginal discharge. We then set off to the hospital.

The contraction I had while in the car was probably one of the worst of all because I couldn't find a position that really helped me cope with it. We were lucky to be one of the only new patients at the maternity ward when we arrived, so we were admitted right away. After the initial check-up, I was glad and relieved to hear that I was already eight centimetres dilated! The nurses broke my water artificially and from then on everything went fast. I felt ashamed to vomit and to have people looking after me, but the staff did a great job. They made us feel at home, everybody was warm and friendly and motivated us a lot. All I had to do was focus on the contractions.

When the baby didn't come out fast enough and his heartbeat started to slow, the doctor decided to use a vacuum to pull the little one out. At that moment I realized that no matter how much I wanted a natural birth with as little intervention as possible I, above all, wanted a healthy baby. Only two hours after arriving at the hospital, Manuel was in our arms. I had expected to cry at this point, but I was just amazed by my little guy. He was so perfect; I was immediately hooked for life.

Unfortunately, the work was not finished. I still had to deliver the placenta, which refused to come out on its own, so the doctor plucked it out piece by piece. For the first time during the delivery I screamed. I definitely wasn't prepared for feeling such serious pain at that point. Manuel was already in his father's arms; the birth should be over, shouldn't it? Well, I had to go through it, and all the pain was gone when I felt Manuel in my arms again. I had lost lots of blood and was pretty weak, but nothing seemed to matter anymore except our little one.

Manuel was born about twenty-five hours after my first contraction, one week past my due date on July 1, 2007, Canada Day, which was quite funny for us, being that we are from Switzerland!

Seeing is Believing
by Jessica Claire Haney

Of all the concerns I had about a successful natural birth—
having strong enough legs to squat for hours, not letting my
emotions or doubts get in my own way, having too small of a
pelvis, and finding out something was wrong with the baby—
breech position never crossed my radar screen. At least, not until
I told my midwife at thirty-four weeks that I felt like I'd been
riding a bike, and the baby seemed lower, which prompted her to
do an internal exam. "You're mostly effaced, but I don't feel any
fontanels," she said. "If that's a butt and not a head, we need to
get this baby to turn."

An ultrasound a week later confirmed my baby was frank
breech (butt down, feet up by his face in pike position). In my
highly litigious area of the United States, the backup doctors for
my birth centre don't allow the midwives to catch breech babies,
so I had to turn the baby around, or be transferred out of the
practice to deliver at the hospital.

It was a good thing that I'd decided to end my teaching job a
month early, as I needed all the extra time to get to chiropractor
and acupuncture appointments, to put my legs above my head,
and to talk to my baby. I told him it was safe to turn, but part of
me stopped believing it was true after our external-version

attempt failed. I'd read that sometimes babies know best, there could be a reason for the position, and I wanted to respect my baby's choice. I could have transferred my care to a solo-practice midwife, but it just didn't feel right. I didn't want my zeal for a natural birth to trump my son's needs.

The doctor who attempted the external version, a lying of hands on the belly to physically turn the baby, is one of the only doctors in my area to happily deliver breech babies vaginally. However, he said that since I was a small-framed, first-time mom with an average-sized (not small) baby, we'd probably end up with a C-section. Still, he respected my desire to try to go as natural as possible, for as long as possible. "Call me when you can't take it anymore," he said, agreeing to let me go into labour on my own.

My blood pressure had other plans. It had been creeping up over the last several weeks of my pregnancy, but since it didn't come with weight gain or terrible swelling I wasn't concerned. No one mentioned that blood pressure alone could be a cause for intervention. I'd been so busy researching tips for turning a breech baby that I didn't give a second thought to the slowly increasing numbers until my forty-week appointment.

Homeopathy had failed to produce the momentum of contractions that I had hoped for, but I told my husband, John, the night before my early Friday-morning appointment that he needed to come too, just in case. I'd been dilated three or four centimetres for more than two weeks and was four days overdue, feeling concerned about my baby getting bigger by the day. It felt like something was ready to shift, but I had no idea it would be in the form of an acronym: PIH. My blood-pressure reading categorized me as having Pregnancy Induced Hypertension. There was no protein in my urine, but the doctor said he couldn't let me go home, and that unless we got a lower reading, I'd have to be induced.

John and I sat back down in the crowded waiting room and waited for the nurse to come check me a third time. When she quietly handed me the small slip of paper with "140/100" written in pencil, I knew I was now bound to the hospital protocol I'd taken Bradley classes to avoid.

When I called the woman we'd hired to be my birth assistant at the birth centre, she was in the middle of a second birth in two days and was unable to join us. I felt given up on, as though there was really nothing she could do for me now that I was out of the safety of the birth centre and was about to be hooked up to a Pitocin drip.

"Do you want me to ask the midwife intern if she can do it?" she asked. The intern had been with me at appointments and had given me advice on using moxibustion to turn the baby. Yes, I needed her there, I said. I needed a connection to what was supposed to have been my experience.

In the parking garage, John and I removed my bags of clothing, essential oils, and organic food from the trunk of my car. He'd driven separately, planning to head off to work after the appointment. Our matching beige cars sat side by side, waiting for us until our lives would be forever changed, when we would come home as a family of three. Rolling a suitcase and toting a blue birth ball, we walked back into Labour and Delivery so I could be admitted and connected to machines. Because of my blood pressure, I was made to lie on my left side in what felt like a defeated position. The monitors showed I was already contracting every seven to ten minutes, though, and I was heartened to think that my body was perhaps marginally ready for action. The doctor had agreed to put me on the lowest possible dose of Pitocin, but even that small amount proved to be more than I could take. My HypnoBirthing strategies went out the window as my contractions double-peaked. By the time I turned on a relaxation CD, I was already so mad at my body for not tolerating the pain that within minutes, I demanded the meditative voice be shut off, and I sent everyone out of the room so I could cry alone. The drugs started to drip into my veins in the late morning, but I made no progress in terms of dilation or the baby's position. By late afternoon, the doctor said, "Well, we can do a C-section now or a C-section later." My midwife intern assured me, "There's no reason you need to rush. Just get the epidural so that you can relax before you face the surgery."

Although I almost went crazy sitting up through a contraction while the anesthesiologist put in the epidural, within minutes I felt like a different person. I could joke and laugh and try to breathe into the reality of having a surgical birth within the next few hours. Gone was the tremendous sense of failure and the anger at everyone who wasn't having my contractions for me. There were still pangs of disappointment and jealousy when the nurse came back after a surprisingly long delay with the report, "Sorry. We've had a busy night. Just had two more babies!" Still, the drugs—given, in part, to counter the pain of the induction of drugs—shifted my entire perspective toward one of acceptance and anticipation of the parenting journey.

When we finally got word after 8:00 p.m. that an OR was

almost ready for us, we asked if we could have another person in the room. For more than two years, I had been working with a craniosacral therapist to help me get healthy enough in mind and body to even get pregnant. I'd come to believe that birth trauma and emotional wounds in my childhood had played a significant role in some of my health struggles. My therapist, Nishanka, worked with children as well as adults and was on board to provide birth support and postpartum care for us. The doctor allowed her into the room and allowed her to videotape the procedure. I didn't know if I would ever watch the video, but I wanted to have it anyway since I wasn't sure what I would see or remember of the procedure.

Nishanka and John dressed in their OR suits, looking to me like HAZMAT inspectors. We'd never taken any C-section prep classes and hadn't done much reading on the subject, so we had little idea what to expect. Nishanka stood at my feet with the camcorder while John sat behind my head. The anesthesiologist suggested to him, "Tell her what's going on." John narrated the movements of the doctors while they twisted my baby boy's bottom and then body out of my abdomen. At 9:30 p.m., Elliott emerged and was moved to the side of the room for cleaning. John came back to me and said through tears and a smile, "He's beautiful. He's perfect."

As far as I was concerned, I could not see the baby fast enough. When Elliott was wrapped and finally brought to me on the table, he took one of my fingers in his right hand and one of John's in his left. We sang to him, "You Are My Sunshine," and he looked at me with startling intensity. Although I wanted desperately to bring him to my breast, I knew he was safe under his father's watch.

When John later joined me in the recovery room without the baby, I was livid. John had wanted to see me, but the nursery staff wasn't ready yet to send in the baby, even though we had requested he receive no bath and no vaccinations. "Get my baby back here!" I shouted. Our nurse, who'd been with us all day and was about to finish her shift, pleaded with the nursery staff over the phone: "This family has gotten nothing they wanted. The mother will do 'skin to skin,' and I'm sure his temperature will rise." Then she turned to the midwife intern from the birth centre and said, "Why don't you go down there and see what you can do."

Soon Elliott was in my arms and nursing. Nishanka did craniosacral therapy and massage on both of us, helping me with my tense, shaking shoulder—a reaction to the anesthetic—and helping Elliott process his birth and unwind his hips. I later learned that breech babies sometimes require hip harnesses because of the stress of having been in the pike position.

I also later learned more about why he had been breech. When I was left alone in the OR, I remembered at almost the last minute to ask, "Can I see the placenta?" We hadn't planned on doing anything with it, but I remembered how impressive it was when I attended my sister's home birth, and I wanted to see what my body had produced. Attached to the beautiful branching sac was a short stub of an umbilical cord. I commented that it looked short, and I later learned it was only about 8 inches long, a third of the normal length. Based on the high position of my placenta and the short length of the cord, a vaginal delivery probably wouldn't have been a safe possibility without risk of the placenta detaching before the baby could be delivered.

I have to believe that this experience, though not what I'd imagined or hoped for, was what my son needed and somehow what I needed, too. It called into question my assumptions about women who "failed" to give birth naturally as having just "not tried hard enough." My initial struggles with breastfeeding, which were probably, in part, a result of the C-section and my stress over it, similarly humbled me and made me more compassionate toward other mothers.

Despite my disappointment and the fact that I think my body was left reeling for months, possibly years, from the chemicals I received in the hospital, and despite my sadness that my son's birth included forceps in the last move to extract his head while keeping his chin to his chest, I am grateful for many aspects of the experience. The first night of my son's life, my husband was allowed to sleep with him on his chest, skin to skin. The second night, I held

Elliott and nursed him on and off all night long with nary a glance from the hospital staff. We cleansed the energy in our room with essential oils, and my doctor allowed me to go home just forty-six hours after my son's birth. "Your next one will be natural," he assured me.

On my son's first birthday, John and I watched the whole surgery and the hour that followed when I was in recovery alone and John was with Elliott. The healing power of having this technology surprised me. Having lived for a year with lingering frustration that my husband had left our son for a few minutes in the nursery, I had the privilege of watching footage that Nishanka took of John hovering over Elliott, keeping him safe from the blinding white lights and assuring him he was loved.

Even if the videotape disintegrates, I will never forget the power of seeing my husband's dedication to our son. Nor will I ever forget seeing my son's first blink and his absorbing look straight into the eyes of the masked surgeon, a kind man who is responsible for a large number of the VBACs (Vaginal Births after Cesarean) in my area. That moment, one that I could not see with my own eyes from behind the green curtain, will forever represent to me hope and openness to the future.

In Her Own Way
by Jill Cunès

My birth story began when I was a medical student. Eight weeks of OB/GYN had galvanized my thoughts and feelings around birth into a few simple resolutions for my own future labour and delivery:

−I would never be an old primigravida.

−I would never have an instrumental delivery (the post-delivery perineum is not pretty from any angle, let alone adding forceps into the equation).

−I would give birth at home, and not under some hospital's labour-and-delivery protocol.

Condition number one required some immediate action on my part, since I considered thirty years to be in the "old" category at that time, and I was getting closer. This is how, four months later, my husband and I set about starting our family. It turns out that only two weeks of "trying" was all it took before he knocked me up.

I walked around feeling stunned and a little nauseous for a week before I organized myself and called the midwife in our neighbourhood. Delivery time? Probably late July, if my dates were right. Forget it, booked up for summer dates. I had the same response from the only other midwifery centre in town. I was told I could try a centre in a nearby city, Ottawa. I pictured myself driving for an hour and a half in active labour, nine months down the road, and figured this was a bad idea from every angle. I cried at my desk, and felt sorry for myself after hanging up the phone. Then, I got over it and called my family doctor, who has an obstetrics practice.

In the end, it didn't really matter who was following me, since I matched to a residency program across the country in Vancouver. At thirty-six weeks pregnant, I showed up for my first day at work. I was having a dream pregnancy and felt great. I even played a little Ultimate Frisbee during the resident-orientation afternoon, hoping it might get things going. What the hell, I thought, I was thirty-eight weeks pregnant by then and that seemed like a great gestational age to give birth.

But at thirty-nine weeks, I was going nowhere fast. I had stopped work and was getting sick of waddling down the street for gelato and iced matcha latte. Where was my baby? Still, I didn't panic. But at my next prenatal checkup, the nurse said, "Uh-oh…looks like your blood pressure is up a little." Never one to have white-coat hypertension, I finally started to worry. My OB wanted to induce me then and there. I resisted. I remember sitting in the delivery suite while working, waiting for the women who had had inductions to actually give birth. Too many ended up in C-section and there was no way I was going to cast my lot with that crowd without a fight. My OB gave me a week to go into labour before she was going to insist, she said.

Six days later, I was desperate. All the tests had been reassuring, but my blood pressure was still up and climbing. My husband phoned his friend who is a homeopath and asked for his advice on what herbs to take. My friend gave me a recipe passed on by her midwives for a castor oil induction. I sipped raspberry-leaf tea to tonify my uterus and tried to send the vibe to my little one that he, she, or it had better decide to come out soon, or else. I failed the castor oil despite hours of wincing and writhing in the bathroom that afternoon, and wound up in the hospital the next morning at 7:00 a.m. for my induction.

In the cubicle next to us, the woman's partner smelled like stale beer and cigarettes. Nothing like a last hurrah the night before your wife pops out a baby, I guess. Our obstetrician showed up, and since my cervix was totally closed, we started with a mechanical dilatation. We returned home and I walked around for a while, contracting a little. After a couple hours, my plug came out and I was at around three centimetres. Back to the hospital.

I had a local prostaglandin application next, which took about a half hour to take effect, but once it did, the party started in full swing. I walked as long as I could, doing laps around the labour and delivery ward. It all seemed fairly benign and amusing until I found myself in the bathroom, no longer able to walk comfortably, feeling like I was going to eject the entire contents of my abdomen into the toilet, and wondering if this is what active labour feels like. I hastily retreated to the labour room, trying to find a comfortable position. There was none to be found, and I panted and moaned, my mom and husband trying to support me through the most intense feelings that I have ever had. I was still adamant about no epidural.

The best relief I could find was to use the precious seconds between contractions to lie back into my husband and clear all the tension and intensity from my body. It was enough to brace me and keep me sufficiently clearheaded to continue. Soon my obstetrician came in. I was about six centimetres dilated and I told her she could rupture my membranes. All I remember is that it was far more uncomfortable than I had anticipated and after that, the contractions and labour are a blur, they happened so fast.

I actually considered asking for an epidural when my worried husband asked the nurse how long this would continue. I was feeling pushy at that point, but they told me, "No, they just checked you; you're definitely not fully dilated yet. The baby will probably be born in another five to six hours." Not pushing was the most difficult task in my life so far. It felt like a tsunami knocking on the door of my cervix while trying to brace it with the muscles of my pelvic floor, which are pretty unimpressive to look at during anatomy class, if you want to know the truth.

At this point, all I could coordinate myself to utter was, "I want to push." I guess the tone in my voice tipped off the labour nurse that I was actually ready. She checked and lo and behold, the signals my body was sending were right on target. Epidural or not, never have I felt such relief to actually be able to direct pain by doing something about it. And I sure did push. No noise, no fuss, just hard work and feeling the results of my efforts.

I was carrying a small baby, I knew after my growth scan the week before. It wouldn't be long before she came out. I was doing it. But suddenly, a rush of people came in, including an obstetrics senior resident and her staff, and the pediatric team, to boot, so I knew things must be looking bad on the monitor. My baby was having decelerations, they told me, and had to come out. I asked what kind, knowing that late decels are the most ominous, but she said "variable," so I focused back on my pushing job. They must have been pretty deep variables, though, because with the next contraction, I was told I was going to get some help. I saw a vacuum extractor come out of the sterile packaging. So much for my non-medicalized birth!

It was amazing to me afterward that I didn't panic in that moment and kept my focus, knowing what the aftermath of a precipitous delivery can look like. I think I didn't have any choice. It had only been five hours of actual labour, but it was time. We were having the baby, and I was ready.

My daughter came out grunting and struggling to breathe, needing a little oxygen to help her get started, but vigorous enough by a minute of life. After being examined by the pediatric team, she was carried over to me, sweetly bundled and looking for something to suck on. A good eater from day one. Sanjay announced her name, Saumya, to everyone. This made us seem like extremely good planners, but actually it was a stroke of luck, as we hadn't been able to agree ahead of time on a boy's name.

The repair of my tear was a difficult task. It took more than half an hour, and was only tolerable because I cuddled the new little life in my arms. No amount of local anesthesia could compensate for the insult of having someone fiddle with my shredded perineum after childbirth. But I didn't care. It was my first lesson about the things we learn to accept for the sake of our kids.

After some delicious peanut-butter toast, they wheeled me to postpartum. I remember saying to somebody, "That wasn't so bad. I could do that again. Not tonight, I mean. Another time."

Pain
by Suzanne Kamata

I was afraid of the pain. Almost from the minute I knew that I was pregnant with twins, I dreaded "the trauma of childbirth." I could handle the three to five months of nausea, the insomnia, the weight gain, even the responsibilities of the next eighteen or so years, but not, I thought, "the most agonizing pain known to mankind."

My sister-in-law in Ohio gave birth to a six pound, twelve ounce boy in two hours with an epidural. "It was almost fun," she told me. "I could feel him coming through the birth canal, but it didn't hurt." She showed me the video: Elton John played on a boom box, her mother bustled about. My brother narrated the event.

"That's what I want, too," I said. Except instead of Elton John, we'd have Enya. There'd be champagne chilling in the mini-fridge. Of course, I'd have the epidural. And my mother wouldn't be in the delivery room—just my husband, Yukiyoshi.

But I live in Japan and no one that I talked to here had ever heard of any kind of anesthesia during normal childbirth. A Japanese friend, who gave birth to a nearly ten-pound baby, was in labour for twenty-four hours with no pain relief. In Japan, I'd heard, a woman in labour was supposed to endure her pain in silence. If she cried out, she'd failed in some way. I vowed to be silent.

Even though they don't use anesthesia, Japanese women have age-old ways of reducing the pain. A small baby makes for an easy delivery and several women gave me advice on restricting the size of my twins.

"You should go for walks," a mother of two told me. "You don't want the babies to get too big."

"Don't let your legs get cold," another woman advised. "Cold legs can lead to a miscarriage." In my fifth month of pregnancy, my mother-in-law announced that it was time for an *obi*, a thick band tied around my waist to keep the babies from getting too large. I was horrified. It sounded worse than Chinese foot-binding. Twins are usually underweight and I didn't want to do anything to impede their growth.

I asked my obstetrician about the practice, just to be polite. I had no intention of wrapping my middle.

"In the old days," he explained, "people had their babies at home. There was no recourse in the event of a difficult birth. They did whatever they could to have an easy labour."

I didn't go for walks. I lazed around on the sofa admiring baby clothes in the Lands' End catalogue. I watched CNN and ABC news on satellite TV. I snuggled under an afghan, keeping my legs warm. And I threw up. And then I started to bleed.

During my hospital stay for a threatened miscarriage, my room was across from the delivery room. I heard women screaming out in the night, "*Itai! Itai! Itai!*" (It hurts! It hurts! It hurts!) and "*Iya! Iya! Iya!*" (No! No! No!) I was terrified. I wondered if it was too late to change my mind.

The doctor recommended cerclage, a procedure in which the cervix is sutured shut to help prevent premature labour. After my first scare, he didn't have to work hard to persuade me.

"Do you want anesthesia?" he asked me. "And if so, what kind?"

He told me that some women went through the operation with no pain relief at all. It sounded brave, but I am a wimp. "Give me the spinal," I said.

Before the operation, I was jabbed with a needle in the arm. When it was time for the epidural, I assumed the fetal pose and waited for the prick in my spine, my delicate spine. In my home country, an anesthesiologist would have handled this part, but there was no one extra here, just the obstetrician and nurses. My mind was haunted by newspaper stories of mixed-up medicines and incompetent doctors. If he missed, would I be paralyzed for life?

I was nude and everyone else was garbed in sterile blue, mouths hidden by ridged masks, only dark eyes visible. They didn't say anything except, "This will hurt." I wanted to ask someone to tell me a story, to distract me with words and questions like my doctor back in South Carolina did.

I felt a cool hand pressing on my thigh, keeping me still for the needle that was about to go in. The first time I flinched a little, but didn't make a sound. It didn't really hurt until the liquid was injected, and then it ached so much that I clenched my jaw.

I heard the doctor sigh. "Sorry. Gotta try it again."

It took two more jabs before the needle was properly inserted. Each time I felt the same ache, but I didn't cry out. Not even a whimper.

I borrowed videos on Lamaze from the hospital. The woman in the first video made it look so easy. She didn't scream, although a few tears trickled down her cheek. The baby slithered right out of her and was suddenly at her breast.

The Lamaze method: Breathe in. Breathe out with the pain. In, out. I practiced. I thought that maybe it wouldn't be so bad after all.

I was surprised by blood again when I was six months pregnant.

"Threatened premature labour," the doctor said, and sent me to bed for the duration.

I was hooked up to an IV and my movements were restricted. I brushed my teeth while on my back and ate my meals at a 45-degree angle. For ten days, my feet did not touch the floor. Even so, my belly continued to tighten with contractions and blood stained the white sheets.

I was transferred by ambulance to another, bigger hospital—one with lots of incubators and a brand new NICU (Neonatal Intensive Care Unit). This time I had roommates—two other women who were expecting twins in July. Mine were due in September.

The other women were there according to hospital policy. Since there is an increased risk of premature labour for multiple pregnancies, women expecting more than one baby are put under observation as a matter of course in the eighth month.

We passed around magazines and brainstormed baby names. We traded snacks and old wives' tales. We worried together about the pain of childbirth. My second night there, we talked about ordering a pizza in a few days. It was like an adult slumber party.

A friend brought me novels. I read all day. Once in a while, a nurse came to monitor the babies' heartbeats. They kicked and squirmed and their hearts were strong.

My parents called each morning from South Carolina and my mother-in-law dropped by with washed pyjamas and cream puffs. My sister-in-law's husband's aunt came by along with a friend of my husband's family. "You shouldn't read," she told me. "It excites the mind and is bad for your baby." She said that I should lie quietly and talk to my babies. For three months.

My husband came every day after teaching high-school physical education and coaching baseball. He brought my mail. One evening, he brought a letter saying that one of my short stories, published the previous fall in a small literary magazine in Illinois, had been chosen by a famous poet for a literary anthology. I couldn't wait to tell my parents.

I was starting to relax. I was even beginning to enjoy myself. The doctor announced that I could start using the toilet again. The catheter was removed and I began testing my shaky legs, taking my first tentative steps toward wellness. Or so I thought.

The next morning, I awoke soaked in blood. My roommates slept through my frantic call to the nurse. Soon, I lay on an operating table awaiting an emergency C-section. I was surrounded by Japanese-speaking strangers wearing blue gauze masks and matching smocks. Yukiyoshi was outside in a waiting room with my wedding ring in his pocket (no jewellery allowed during surgery). The rest of my family was thousands of miles away. I had lived in Japan for ten years, but it had never felt as foreign as it did at that moment.

"*Itai, itai, itai,*" I said. I'd gone through thirty minutes of labour and already my vow of silence was shattered. I was secretly impressed, however, by my ability to communicate in a foreign language under such extreme circumstances.

I'd expected everything to be different. I'd expected ice cubes in my mouth and my husband's fingers kneading my lower back. Instead, I was clutching the hand of a stranger and I was scared.

Someone told me to curl up in a ball. I eased onto my side and curled. I felt the needle slide into my spine, but this time it didn't hurt at all. My lower body became warm and then went quickly numb.

The obstetrician started swabbing my middle with antiseptic. Another man, identified as the neonatal specialist, entered the room. "Twenty-six-week baby very difficult," he told me in heavily accented English. "I will do my best."

I looked at the clock. It was 8:30 a.m. I didn't want to think about what was going to happen in the hours, days, weeks to follow.

I was sorry that I'd ever wished for an easy birth. With a few extra weeks in the womb, my babies' lungs would have fully developed. They'd have had enough fat on their bodies to maintain the proper temperature. They would have received vital antibodies and nutrients through the placenta. These gifts of the body made my fear of physical pain seem petty.

Minutes later, the obstetrician sliced open my abdomen and pulled out my son. I couldn't see what was happening because a screen had been set up over my chest, but I could feel the liquid ooze over my belly and the fishlike squirm of my 964-gram baby boy. "*Kawaii*," the nurse holding my hand said. "He's cute." I heard his cry—a tiny mewling—and then he was whisked away.

"Now we'll go in for the other one," the doctor said. He quickly delivered my 690-gram daughter, the one who had lived beneath my heart for six and a half months. And then she was gone, too.

I lay on the table, resigned and passive. This was supposed to be one of the most joyous moments of my life, but I felt like a failure. Although I'd tried to do the right thing throughout—abstaining from coffee and alcohol, avoiding travel and smoky rooms—there was a chance that my babies wouldn't make it through the day.

Because I was recovering from surgery, I didn't see my children for twenty-four hours. My husband was allowed into the NICU and he reported back to me. "They're cute," he said, "but not like that." He pointed to the babies on the cover of one of my books. "They look like little baby birds."

The following evening, I was wheeled to the NICU and I saw my children for the first time. Their bodies were scrawny and red, but they had all ten fingers and toes. I couldn't see their eyes because they were fused shut. They had dark hair on their heads and soft hairs on their shoulders and faces. They both had little beards.

The neonatal specialist told me that although there were many hurdles ahead, the babies were doing incredibly well. "Don't worry," he said. "Trust me."

When I was well enough to walk again, I joined the other expectant and new mothers at the dining-room table. My former roommates were eager for details. "Did it hurt?" they asked me.

"No, not at all," I said. And I was disappointed that I'd missed out on the pain.

Finding the Way
by Laura Johnson Dahlke

Giving birth is like voyaging through a portal to another world. You can't see exactly what's ahead of you and you can't go back once your odyssey begins. Once labour moves to a certain point, you're in—you're *all* in—with your baggage dragging at your feet and a mind amuck with travel plans.

I went through that portal a second time almost a year ago with my husband, daughter, midwife, two nurses and my determination. I gave birth after three hours of desperately difficult labour. I wouldn't wish my second labour on anyone. Here and now, I retract my former optimism about drug-free birth. It's hard as nails. No mistake.

When my daughter Julia was born more than eight years ago, Eileithyia, the goddess of childbirth, must have been watching out for me. It was a positive, transformative experience; a manageable toil that ended after six hours. It was a textbook drug-free labour and delivery, through which I never felt desperate. Julia's birth made me believe in natural childbirth and while challenging, it was never overwhelming. After she arrived, I felt so accomplished and positive about birth that I wanted to share my experience with other women. I would say, "It's not so bad. You can do it drug-free, too."

Well, I got my payback. I got my ass kicked during my son Phineas's birth. If I ever said, "It's not so bad," to you and you wanted to smack me, I now understand why. Sorry.

So, here's what happened.

I had hard, hard labour from the onset, because I was already dilated five centimetres when I started. I was experiencing tsunami-intense contractions that lasted and lasted. Once I arrived at the birth centre my seasoned, gray-haired midwife, Roberta, broke my waters. I was later told that inducing labour this way could cause more acute labour pains. Yeah, I'll vouch for that.

When I was at nine and a half centimeters, the contractions were so difficult that I "grayed out." I went somewhere else, somewhere far, far away from those contractions and that homey room at the birth centre. I went far away from my husband Josh's medical residency, our lonely lives in San Diego, my need to have a mothering mother. I went far away from that outrageous pain on my cervix. It was a mini-vacation that I now see as one of this birth's lessons: Get out of your own way and ask for help.

During the time that I was "grayed out," the video footage shows me lying on my side with my husband talking to me, stroking my hair and being an attentive, knowledgeable doula. He was helping me move through the portal and as best he could, trying to ease my suffering. Our lives in San Diego had been arduous—he was in his OB/GYN Residency at the Naval Medical Center with our families and friends in the Midwest. We had no support. Josh often worked eighty or more hours a week and harder than most could know. He sometimes worked merciless twenty-four-hour shifts and was then expected to drive to local hospitals to do patient rounds. He'd come home and collapse into bed. Exhaustion is not even the word.

I took care of Julia, paid bills, cooked, shopped, cleaned, did laundry, did yoga, got oil changes, finished my second master's degree, started teaching at the college level, and saw to every last detail of our lives. We were crazy busy and alone. During Phineas's birth, my husband was present and helpful and offered the support I sorely lacked during the last four years.

But, in this moment during labour, I still thought I had to do it all. Because of this, I subconsciously made up my mind that I didn't want help; I could manage. Well, that's nonsense. I can see now that I needed all of the succor I could get and my son's birth helped bring me to that awareness.

While my daughter's birth was painful, it wasn't suffering. That purposeful pain opened me up and sent endorphins through my body. After her delivery, I'd never felt such exuberant joy. But during Phineas's birth, I suffered. I couldn't relax, try as I did. The contractions came on stronger and longer, stronger and longer, and I breathed deep, trying to move out of the way and endure. I stayed quiet. I was trying to keep myself together like I'd been able to do during Julia's birth.

While sitting upright in the Jacuzzi, holding on to the sides and not leaning back, Roberta told me, "The water will hold you. Let it." But I couldn't. She also suggested my husband get in the tub with me. "Let him support your legs." But I wouldn't have it. I just sat on edge and tried to go to a deep place, knowing my thighs and butt ached and were in need of support. Breathing. Internalizing. Trying to do it on my own.

I was tough. I was solid. I was in the worst pain in my life, and

I couldn't call out, "Help me!" I couldn't scream, "Fuck this!" I just couldn't let myself go, so my body let go for me. But needing your mind to go gray just so you can accept help is no way to labour, or to live. I halted at nine and a half centimetres.

Racked with pain and the inability to push past it, I clung to the edge at nine and a half centimetres. I looked at my midwife from that cliff and said, "My daughter's birth wasn't like this. Nothing helps!" She had me move onto my side, "dangle" in my husband's arms, rock, sit on the toilet. You name it, we were trying it, and yet I couldn't reach "complete." I can't begin to describe that tedious pain. So, I rocked and swayed and moaned and got onto all fours staying with it, staying with it. Apparently, Phineas's head needed to flex. Rock, sway, moan, every fibre of my body, my uterus.

While I was on all fours, Roberta decided to intervene. "Just let me hold the cervix back while you push," she encouraged. "Can you try that?"

I nodded, looking in her eyes the way women in labour look at their midwives—searching for acknowledgement, direction, and understanding. Crouched at my feet, she looked fully at me with kind, grandmotherly eyes. She knew all about this pain I was feeling; she had three children of her own and had been a midwife for more than forty years. Yes, I could try it. I trusted her completely. Roberta put on a sterile glove, moistened it with jelly, and held back my cervix while I pushed. Together we made it disappear.

"It's gone," she said after one push, relieved and smiling. My cervix was gone.

My body needed time to catch up with itself. In two and a half hours I'd gone from five centimetres to complete, and my body needed a moment to gather energy and synthesize labour before delivery. In this latency phase of the second stage of labour, I rested as the contractions eased. I ate honey, drank vitamin C, and breathed. I was ready to continue.

Pushing was deep and awkward. In both of my children's births, I never had the urge to push; it was a conscious effort. So, I pushed and made progress without that guide. For about half an hour, I pushed and waited and pushed more. This was tiring but not as painful as before. Then, it burned and stung. How was I going to do this? I've heard it said that all births reach this point: between a rock and a hard place. If nine and a half centimetres had not been this place, then it was, most certainly, arriving at the crowning phase.

Crowning is a remarkable moment both as the start of the child's final journey from nascency to independent life and for its behemoth pain. With my legs in two nurses' arms, my midwife waiting to catch, my daughter and husband cheering me on, I pushed without wanting to push.

I talked to myself, "How can I do this? How am I going to do this? I can't do this." "Yes you can!" everyone shouted around me. So, I pushed in the way someone might if they were going to knife themselves. I thrust into the push, and all the pain that went with it, just to finish the job.

"Is the head out?" I wanted to know. It was. At this point, it became important to get the baby out in less than a minute. So, I pushed without a contraction. I waited for another contraction but it didn't come.

"We need to get the baby out now, Laura," Roberta said

seriously. I understood but nothing was happening. Without another try, she rolled me on my side to apply downward pressure on his head. Yet again, I required assistance to complete the crossing into that other world. Finally, his blood- and mucous-covered body emerged from me. Our parting had been a quick but gruelling miracle.

Phineas was born on May 19th at 11:35 p.m. after three short hours, but one overwhelmingly painful passage. On that warm San Diego evening, we greeted our son. I was dazed and shaking after the delivery, but in awe of his beauty.

"Maybe we should try this the pain-free way next time," Josh said with exhaustion. I thought he might be right.

About an hour after the birth, I thanked the nurses and midwife for helping me. I meant it completely and in a way I've never known before. I was utterly open and grateful. I knew I had needed their support and guidance as I walked through the portal of pregnancy to delivery. They were there and I had needed them.

"It's all you. You delivered the baby," Roberta said. But I knew she had intervened at important intersections; she'd been the shaman ushering the way. The nurses examined Phineas and then let us rest. We were doing well, and five hours later we went home. Going home put us all at an advantage. We normalized quickly and I was able to rest comfortably.

It would be a long time before I'd want to relive the birth. It would be even longer before I might understand that my suffering had guided me toward seeking and enjoying assistance, and that being connected to others and depending on them was an enlightened surrender.

"Yes, you can," they had told me. And so, I did.

Cohen's Birth Story
by Chelsie Anderson

I woke up on Saturday feeling the same as always: uncomfortably pregnant and optimistic that today would be the day! Mali and Kale, our three and one year olds, had spent the previous night with Nana, so we were able to sleep in a bit and lounge around. It being the day after baby's due date, I was feeling eager to say the least. I had spent the last few days taking herbs (black and blue cohosh) hoping to get things started, and trying to remember what my midwife Nadine had said, "The herbs will only work if baby is ready to come anyway." *Don't be so anxious* had become my mantra during the past few weeks, yet I couldn't help but take the herbs, but to no avail. My baby was clearly in no rush to greet the world.

The day was beautiful, it was Saturday and we were kid-free, so I suggested to my husband, Scotty, we go for a walk and a coffee. I announced over coffee that I'd be having our baby later in the day; I figured with positive words the baby would surely come. I guess I'd been crying wolf for too long though, as Scotty borrowed a movie he was certain he'd watch that night despite my announcement. *Argh*, I was sure this baby would have come by now! My first two babies were born two weeks before their due dates, therefore, making it to forty weeks seemed like too much hard work.

So, we walked home. No contractions, not even any little cramps. I was begging to feel something, just to have some confirmation that this baby would arrive soon. How long could one be pregnant in the middle of as hot a summer as this one had been? The only outfit that fit, a borrowed dress I'd been wearing for two months solid, was getting tired, or at least I was tired of it.

The walk had wiped me out even though it had only taken twenty minutes. So, I went to lie down, after which we tried another "natural induction" method. Semen is apparently full of prostaglandins that can induce labour. From this time onward I felt decidedly "heavy" and tired. The baby felt low, and my uterus felt weighed down. The thought of going on another walk, as we were planning, seemed horrendous. All I could do at that moment was sit in the living room with *Macleans* and read articles that seemed all too unimportant. I couldn't focus on the articles, as my body was demanding attention. What I was feeling? I couldn't quite decipher the sensations. Was something different, or was I just wishing for something to be different? I was trying so hard to feel something, what was it? Scotty came in from mowing the lawn and was set to head back out again, but the thought of him leaving made me uncomfortable. I made him grab the cell phone on his way out the door.

"But I'll just be out back!" he said. I grabbed our landline and went to lie down in bed with my magazine. Again, I was struggling to focus on the words. After reading the same sentence about eight times I finally admitted defeat, put it down, and closed my eyes. I immediately opened them again to help me focus on the tiniest sensation. "Was that a bit of a backache?" Not sure. I decided to call Scotty; it would be nice to have him nearby.

By the time I dialed his number and he answered I was suddenly certain that I needed him immediately. I called desperately into the phone, "Mate, come in."

"Really?"

Click, I hung up. It was too distracting to be holding the phone.

Oooh, a contraction. Hurry Scotty…

Shit, another one. Where is he? I finally heard him run up the front steps. I paged the midwives, or at least I thought I had.

"Can you fill the tub?" I called out. He was already on it, connecting pipes to taps, etcetera. We'd been through the drill. Our baby was to be born into a kiddie pool, which we'd had inflated for weeks in our bedroom.

Another contraction. I practiced breathing through floppy lips and thought about *Spiritual Midwifery*. What would Ina May say now? I momentarily pondered this thought while Scotty madly raced around. I had decided ahead of time that water imagery might be helpful during the contractions, so I was trying to focus on waves crashing over my body, and just being part of it all.

I paged the midwives again. Why hadn't they called back? It seemed like an eternity had passed since the first page. Another contraction. I moaned this time and asked Scotty for the hot water bottle. He called back, "Do you want hot tap water or boiling water?"

I refused to answer. I had to focus. My thought space seemed limited; surely he could work it out. I paged the midwives again.

When Scotty returned to the room, I asked about the tub and he said it was ready whenever I was. Up until that point I'd been lying as still as possible on the bed, trying to hold the baby back until the midwives arrived. I wasn't prepared for an unattended birth. With the next contraction I pooped. "*Quelle horreur!*" I confessed to Scotty, feeling humiliated as he cleaned me; what a champ! He left the room, and when he came back he sounded uneasy. In a wavering voice he said, "Chels you'd better get into the tub, I think I can see the baby."

I didn't respond. Moving seemed like an impossible request at that moment.

With the next contraction I felt revitalized and what needed to be done was suddenly clear.

"Mate, you know what to do," I said.

Both Nadine and Jane, our fabulous midwives, had been through the "how to deliver a baby" speech with us in previous weeks, and he was going to have to remember his training! I needed him to feel confident in his abilities so that he could help me to feel the same. It was becoming obvious we were going to do this on our own. I asked Scotty to check the midwives' pager number for me. He paged.

Suddenly determined to get me in the tub, Scotty pushed it—full of water and all squishy as it was a blow-up one—all the way to the edge of the bed: what a superhero! He gave me a brief motivational speech. It worked, and before my next contraction I somehow stepped off the bed, and swung my legs and body over the edge of the tub. Bliss! The warm water felt so good! I trusted it, and relaxed into it.

Jane called back within seconds of Scotty paging. Hallelujah! I was pushing for the first time while he was on the phone. Jane immediately recognized the noises in the background and was on her way. I was on my knees with my head and arms resting on the edge of the pool. It felt so good and so natural to be in the water; my body felt buoyant and I could focus on its warmth rather than on the birthing sensations. I felt like I was having a big baby, but it didn't concern me, as the water was comforting. Scotty could definitely see the head now and told me so. I could feel the baby almost crown then recede slightly over the next two contractions. On the next push I decided it was time to meet our baby. Scotty was in position. The head came out in one push, then the shoulders and body on the next. My best mate gently slid our little guy up and out of the water. Wow! We suddenly had a baby!

Because the umbilical cord and placenta were still attached, it was a bit of a struggle to flip myself around, but I managed, and quickly—I couldn't wait to see my baby. Scotty put him on my chest, and said he thought it was a boy, but neither of us wanted to check again, as we didn't want to disturb our little buddy. The three of us were elated and amazed at what we'd just accomplished.

"Get the video camera!" We were hoping to film the birth, but clearly, it was too late for that. Instead Scotty filmed the moments just after birth.

"Get the digital camera! Oh yeah, get him a blanket and a hat! Is he cold?"

Little Cohen looked perfect; pink and beautiful. He looked up at me and smiled—I'm sure this happened! After a few more minutes in this euphoric state of almost disbelief Jane and Nadine, our midwives, ran up the front steps at exactly the same time. As they walked in Cohen greeted them with his first big cry, just to let them know he had arrived and was okay.

Jane and Nadine were awesome. Cooing and praising little Cohen, they told us we did great and we looked good, which is how I felt despite the blood-and-guts bath I was taking. I couldn't help but wonder what things would have been like had the paramedics arrived on the scene instead. Thank goodness for midwives, for instilling confidence in us and telling us the birth of a baby is a normal, natural and manageable event. There we were, everyone was happy and doing well, our midwives were calm, telling us that everything was good.

They had arrived just in time for all the "dirty work" of delivering the placenta and putting up with my whining. Having a baby is one thing, but having a placenta is completely different. There's nothing to look forward to at this stage, and I was bleeding quite a bit and feeling shaky. The placenta came out all squishy; it was a good feeling to be rid of it, I felt light again. I had help getting back onto the bed and started calling all the relatives. What a day! My total time in labour, we guessed, must have been about 40 minutes from start to finish, which was half the time of my second baby's birth, which was half the time of my first. Cohen weighed 9 pounds, 6 ounces at birth and was gorgeous!

Cohen's Birth
by Scott Clayton

At 6:03 p.m., Chels called me and said, trembling a little, "Mate, come in." By about 6:10 I could see a five-millimetre crescent of the head and thought the baby must be very close. Chels had called, and was continuing to call, the midwives with no reply. I also tried at about 6:20. At the pager's prompt we had been saying our home number, but after dialing again at 6:28, I realized the prompt was asking us to enter the number.

Jane rang back two minutes later and I said, "Jane we're on."

"Who is this?" she asked.

"Scott and Chelsie."

"Leaving now."

After I spoke to Jane, Chels was concerned that the midwives wouldn't make it in time for the birth. I was also concerned as I could still see the head. I firmly told her that she had to get into the pool between contractions. She moved slowly but positively for the tub and got into a hands-and-knees position. After approximately three contractions, Chels could feel the baby's head was coming!

"Get low in the water," I reminded her. I recalled what the midwives had told us to do: "Make sure the baby is fully submerged at birth, then quickly pull him up and out of the water once born."

Our baby's head "popped" out, facing up, and he looked like he was asleep, absolutely still. Concerned but not panicking, I stared at his face, while reminding Chels to stay low and keep the baby under the water. I stared and stared and I finally noticed small blinking motions. His mouth moved slowly, but remained mostly in a relaxed open position. Since the head had appeared I had my hand under it to support it, and kept my eyes on the baby's face for about ten seconds. Chels pushed one more time. The push took our baby past the bum and I easily guided the rest out and up above the surface. "It's a little boy; we have another little boy!" It was 6:40 p.m. He looked surprisingly perfect, like he was already bathed and well-adjusted to his surroundings. It seemed as if he were sleeping, squinting on occasion, but making no sounds.

Jane and Nadine arrived about five to ten minutes after his birth. I greeted them from the front landing as they bolted across the lawn, gear in hand. Baby had started to cry, and Jane and Nadine heard him as they ran up the front steps.

"Do we have a baby?"

"Yep," I replied casually, as I knew all was well.

The Last Card
by Erica Etelson

Propped up in a bed in the maternity ward, a photo I had seen months before in a midwifery book made an unwelcome appearance in my mind's eye. In it, a joyful couple cuddled at home with their just-born baby. The caption read, "Being with our new baby together renewed our bond of love for one another—we were like newlyweds again." The only newlyweds David and I resembled were Alice and Ralph Kramden, so far were we from the picture of postpartum romantic bliss. What had led us astray? Was it the fluorescent lighting? The nursing pillow strapped around David's waist like a tutu? The catheter in my urethra? Why were we in a hospital at all instead of at home as planned? Nothing that happened before, during, or after the birth of my son conformed to plan. Labour was a primal lesson in surrendering to what I could not control. It was not a lesson I was grateful for, nor did I heed it with anything akin to grace. Being a lawyer, I was anxious to find someone to blame: David, the obstetrician, the reluctant fetus, myself. Blame was a way to regain the illusion of control.

It is true what most counsel, that when it comes to birth outcomes, there is only one thing that really matters. But, it is equally true that every excruciating minute of labour matters and everything that goes awry matters, in a less consequential, but no less enduring, way. In the end, even if your baby is robust and adorable, even if she has the visage of Sophia Loren and is clearly endowed with great intelligence and charm, it is still not easy to let go of the trauma of a difficult birth.

On the first night of our home-birth class it dawned on me that the baby inside me was soon going to hatch and that I was likely to be in a state of consciousness when this happened. Until this point, I had convinced myself that the pain couldn't be as extreme as rumoured, or the human race would have been long since extinct. Could childbirth be more painful than having your leg torn off by a shark, or being burned at the stake, or having your eyes scoured with lye? Such were the warmhearted, maternal thoughts that filled my head as the second trimester unfolded ominously into the third.

When I entered the softly lit room full of couples reclining on pillows, all of whom were there to spend six weeks learning how to help the woman bear the agony of natural childbirth, I began to get nervous. I had decided on a home birth early on, not because I am even remotely brave in the face of pain, but because I had done enough reading to conclude that home-birth outcomes were better for mother and for baby. I was wary of the usually unnecessary medical interventions routinely performed during hospital births: IV drips, vacuum extractions, the dreaded episiotomies and, worst of all, in 250 percent of hospital births, Cesarean sections. I was also convinced that epidurals posed risks to the baby and had heard that labour nurses often encouraged labouring women to end their suffering. Midwives, on the other hand, do not and in fact cannot administer epidurals. If I were in the kind of pain I had heard tale of and was offered waist-down numbness instead, would I take it? Can fish swim?

Instead of drugs, we would have at our disposal alternative pain-management techniques, which we practiced while clenching ice cubes inside our fists. Our options included: breathing deeply, floating away from pain, saying hello to pain, becoming one with pain, saying "fuck you" to pain, as well as grunting, chanting, screaming, moaning, singing, crying, verbally abusing our mates, and sitting in lukewarm birthing tubs which, it was said, could reduce the pain by as much as half. David and I hatched a plan that involved my floating in a tub while he employed guided imagery to hypnotize me into believing I was snorkeling in tropical waters.

On the last night of our class, the instructor gave each couple ten cards. On each card we wrote a desired feature or outcome of our upcoming labours. These were mostly frivolous wishes that revealed our collective naïveté: candlelight, Enya, blueberries, massage, hand-holding. For many of us, our vision of labour looked more like a third date than like the bloody, sweaty, fecal scene of a birth. All the couples had one card in common: healthy mommy, healthy baby. We laid out our ten cards in front of us and one by one turned over the cards in reverse order of relative importance, healthy mommy and baby of course being the last card. Then, the class was over, and we all filed carefully down the stairs and out into the still, August night.

It was my due date, and I was on my way to my parents' hotel when my foot rocked off the side of my clog and I fell forward, landing on hands and knees on the pavement. My knees were scraped and bruised and one of my ribs felt even more tweaked than usual, but that was all. That night as I lay in bed reading, my ankle turned purple and started swelling. When I tried to stand, I winced and plopped back down on the bed, where I would remain for the next two days monitoring my early labour signs and praying that my ankle would un-wrench itself before I went into labour. During the night, I woke up my usual four or five times to pee, but had to do it by standing on one leg, over a bucket beside the bed. To accomplish this, I leaned heavily on David. David assured me that while supporting me was a strain on his legs and groin, he could manage. The next morning David woke up with what was diagnosed that afternoon as an inguinal hernia. He could barely walk.

We were ready to birth our baby.

Four days later, I woke up at 1:00 in the morning feeling like I had to defecate. When I sat on the toilet, I felt cramped and constipated. I went back to bed. Fifteen minutes later, I limped to the toilet with more cramps. Again, no luck. I lay in bed wondering if I could be in labour. No, I didn't think so. Here I was, four days past my due date having intermittent abdominal cramps. No, definitely not labour.

For the third time, I rolled out of bed to go to the bathroom. As I stood up, I felt a trickle of warm water running down my legs. My water had broken, but I was still convinced I wasn't in labour. It didn't feel like labour. It felt more like the time I was in Guatemala and hadn't pooped for four days. In an abundance of caution, I woke up David.

"Your water broke?" He said, sounding sleepy and confused. In our class, we had learned that the water usually doesn't break until well into labour, sometimes not even until the baby pops out.

"I think so," I said. "Yeah, what else could it be?"

"Well then, let's call the midwives," he said.

"I hate to wake them up in the middle of the night if I'm not sure I'm in labour."

"Erica, your water broke. You're in labour. I'm calling."

He went downstairs for their phone number. By the time he was back, the first undeniable contraction had seized me. It was short, mild and unpleasant. It was about as much pain as I thought I could bear.

Our midwife Laurel, on the line with David, reminded him that early labour in a first-time birth would be long and slow, sometimes lasting days, and that we should try if at all possible to get some sleep. She said we should call her again when the contractions were three minutes apart. Three minutes later, we called her back. I groaned into the receiver a few times and handed David the phone. Laurel told him she was on her way.

She arrived forty minutes later, by which time I had already vomited my mother's salmon croquettes into the handy pee bucket beside the bed and was out of my mind with pain. The contractions were coming every two minutes and lasting forty-five seconds. My friend Rose came over as planned to fill up the "Aqua Doula" birthing tub. It took an hour to fill, an hour I spent pacing the hall, glaring resentfully at the Aqua Doula and, every two minutes, letting out a high-decibel bellow as another contraction ripped through me.

Contractions have been described in many ways. Our midwives said they were like *really* bad menstrual cramps. My friend Susan couldn't describe the sensation, but said the pain was the equivalent of pounding your thumb with a hammer again and again. My contractions felt like a bomb exploding in slow motion in my uterus. As a contraction began, my first impulse was to run, to get out of and away from my body. As it intensified to the point where it became clear that escape was impossible, groans and screams came roaring out of me, utterly primal and out of control. Way, *way* out of control.

The best part of a contraction is its denouement; just after it peaks and you know the worst is over, that it will soon end and that you will have up to a minute of rest before it begins again. There's a lot to look forward to during that one-minute interval, such as cold compresses, sips of water, and the amazingly wonderful feeling of not being in agony.

By around five in the morning, my midwives decided that my cervix had opened enough that I was allowed to sit in the birthing tub. The danger of getting into the tub too soon is that labour may slow down. Furthermore, once the water breaks, the clock starts ticking and, according to most practitioners' standards, the baby has to be born within eighteen hours one way or another, vaginally or surgically, because the risk of infection without the protective amniotic sac sealing in the baby becomes too high.

The Aqua Doula was set up in our small, terracotta-tiled sunroom upstairs. The room had ceiling-to-floor windows and a skylight but, in the middle of the night with only a dim light filtering in from the hallway, it felt appropriately cavelike.

At last, I thought as I heaved myself into the tub, 50 percent pain reduction here I come. As the first contraction in the tub began rumbling, I leaned over the edge, gripping its rubbery edge, unsure whether to climb out or stay put. As the contraction subsided, Rose pressed a cold compress to my forehead and held out a cup of water for me to sip through a straw. "This tub isn't all it was cracked up to be," I said. These were my last words for hours. Now and then, the idea that I should pretend to be floating in the ocean in Hawaii crossed my mind. Just float away from bodily sensation, just float away. But with the onset of each new contraction, I was immediately on my hands and knees, bearing down onto the side of the tub and roaring.

David was in the tub with me, or kneeling beside it for most of this time, alternately rubbing my back and trying to stay out of my way. I asked for my special womb-music tape to be played, and this deep, echoing, rhythmic, beating sound is what eventually led me into that place where communication becomes impossible, where labour has gone past the point of tolerance and into the realm of other worldliness, where the woman is the uterus, the uterus is pain, and there's nothing else.

Laurel's cell phone rang and she stepped out of the room. She came back to tell me that another one of her clients had just gone into labour and, like me, was starting fast and furious. She would have to go attend her while Jade stayed with me. Another midwife would be called to back up Jade—did I have any preference as to whom this might be? I stared blankly at Laurel and Jade and shook my head. I didn't care if the Incredible Hulk came to assist at that point.

David climbed into the tub with me again. "It's like snorkeling in Maui, right Erica? Just pretend you're snorkeling." I was unresponsive, and his suggestion fell to the tile floor with a thud as Jade and Rose looked at him like he was insane. "Why don't you take a break, David?" Jade said kindly. "Go down to the kitchen and eat something, it's almost morning."

Another midwife, named Martha, arrived. At some point I looked up from the water where I had been admiring the blood clots floating on the surface and there she was, smiling supportively at me while Jade briefed her on my progress.

As the sky began to lighten, the room began to feel too warm and too bright. I imagined myself spending the entire day in the tub and watching the sun rise again the next morning. That's when my back exploded. I had heard about back labour—when the baby turns face up so that the hard back of its head puts pressure on the mother's spine. It's considered the most painful form of labour and what I most dreaded.

"My back, oh my God, my back!" I shrieked.

"Let me check you," said Jade.

She climbed into the tub with me. Only a home-birth midwife would step into a warm tub full of blood clots and various other bodily fluids. She reached inside me.

"The baby hasn't turned face up, but I think you should get out of the tub now," she said. "You haven't progressed at all in the time you've been in here. I think you need to walk around for a while."

I said that no, I didn't think that was what I wanted to do, thank you very much. Not that the Aqua Doula was such a great place to be after all, but what if it were worse on the outside—it wasn't a chance I could take.

Jade had heard it all before. "You really need to get out now. You don't want to go on and on like this, right? We want to get this over with, especially since your water's already broken."

Rose and Jade nodded. David had at some point slipped back

into the tub unnoticed by me, and he helped me stand up and climb out.

I began pacing the hallway, and the novelty of being upright lifted my spirits, for about twenty seconds. But then my back reclaimed all of my attention. Martha suggested a hot shower. I was thinking more along the lines of a near-lethal dose of morphine, but I cooperatively staggered into the bathroom and got on my hands and knees in the shower. For a few minutes, I stayed there, the hot water blasting down my back until I started feeling dizzy with heat.

"I need to lie down," I announced. I knew that lying down was a frowned-upon activity for mothers labouring at home. Lying down was a counterproductive, conventional, patriarchal labour position that robbed the woman of her power and required the baby to defy gravity to be born, but my bed with its Indian bedspread and flannel pillowcases beckoned me. If only I could crawl into bed, pick up a good book, and pretend that none of this was happening. I lay on my side, one leg propped up on a pillow, and rode out a few contractions in this position. The contractions were now at barely measurable intervals. It was more like one long rolling contraction.

At 11:00 a.m,. I sat up and said that I had had enough. "I want drugs and I want them now," I said, giving David a defiant look.

"Whatever you want, Erica—you know I'm cool with that," he said.

I expected Jade and Martha to be crestfallen—a hospital transport must feel like such a failure to them, but they were unfazed. Jade explained that I could, of course, be transported if I wanted to, but that I was probably very close and that if I hung on a little longer I could probably birth my baby at home. She also said that by the time we drove to the hospital, checked in, got prepped for the epidural and waited for it to take effect, it would be two hours before I felt any relief. She and Martha agreed that if I stayed home, chances were my baby would be born in that same amount of time.

"How about if I check you one more time before you decide?" she said. She reached inside me as I lay there trying to absorb the shocking news that relief was two hours away.

"You're fully dilated," she said. "There's a small flap covering your cervix, but that can be pushed out of the way. It's time to start pushing. Now is not a good time to transport."

So, I started pushing, although I didn't feel that intense urge to bear down that many women describe. On the contrary, I felt as if I didn't understand what the pushing was all about. It was still all I could do to ride out the contraction, and now I had something else to do too, something that I had never done before and didn't know how to do. Had we covered pushing in our class? We had practiced being in a lot of pushing positions like squatting, kneeling, standing, and leaning. We had also learned about the timing of pushing, and how the effort was best expended at the peak of the contraction so as to harness the force of the uterine muscle, but what about the act of pushing itself? I remembered the instructor comparing this final stage of birth to squeezing toothpaste out of the tube. And I remembered that my friend referred to pushing as "shitting a watermelon." Neither metaphor turned out to be particularly helpful.

I hung on David's neck and pushed; the only thing that was squeezed out was a little bit more of David's intestine into his groin. I straddled the toilet backward and pushed. The midwives assured me that a surprising number of babies had been safely birthed over toilets. Rose brought in a tall stack of books and had me prop up one foot on them.

"See, your law books finally came in handy for something," she said, and I actually laughed.

I laughed because I thought the baby was coming soon and I was beginning to feel a bit euphoric. The midwives were clearly in baby-catching mode and David was next to them, ready to catch the baby if they gave him the last-minute okay. Martha held a mirror between my legs so I could see the baby come through. There were quilted sterile pads laid out below me, and the receiving blankets were tumbling in the dryer, ready to envelop the shivering infant.

"I feel the head," said Jade. There was another burst of activity in the bedroom as I squatted next to the bed, holding on to the wood frame and wringing out my final pushes. I started thinking about the "ring of fire"—the final and most intense stage of childbirth when the head comes through, shredding vaginal tissue here and there. It was going to happen any moment now and I no longer feared it because then this would all be over.

Two hours had passed since the time I had declared my transport order. The baby wasn't out. I pushed out some inhuman-smelling feces and the fumes filled the room as Martha, like an angel, silently wiped the tiny pile of poo off the floor and disposed of it. Jade had me push a few more times while she held aside the cervical flap, in case it was that thin bit of flesh that was holding the baby back.

"This isn't working," she said. She and Martha left the room to confer while I lay on the bed in despair, Rose stroking my arm and back.

"I need drugs," I moaned.

"Yes, you do," she said, refraining from reminding me that she had believed all along I would need an epidural.

"I need drugs *now*," I bellowed.

Rose continued stroking my back as though I were part mental patient, part wounded kitten. When the midwives came back in to the bedroom, I announced with all the clarity I could muster, lest my request be misunderstood and hence delayed by an agonizing second, "I need an epidural or a C-section. Now!"

To my amazement, Jade nodded her head in something close to agreement. She wasn't going to check me and she wasn't going to remind me of the evils that lay in wait at the hospital. "Is that your final decision?" she asked.

"Yes!" I screeched as another landmine blew me apart. As the contraction subsided, I added, "And I'm not walking down the stairs. I want to be carried out on a stretcher."

I'm not proud of this moment. This was the all-time low point of my labour, the moment where I couldn't find an ounce of strength to go on, and just wanted that baby out of my body one way or another. I had worked long and hard enough and somehow the thought of staggering down the stairs seemed, after all I'd been through, utterly unthinkable, impossible, the hardest thing anyone could ever ask of me.

To my dismay, Jade sighed heavily. "You can have a stretcher if you want, but you need to understand what's going to happen if we call the paramedics. First of all, they're going to come barrelling in here like there's a full-on emergency. Then, they're going to take complete control. They'll rush you to the hospital where you'll be treated like an emergency labour gone bad, even though that's not what's happening…you know that's not what's happening, right?"

I nodded mournfully.

"So, it's totally your decision of course. I'll call 911 if you want. Why don't you take a few minutes by yourself to decide." Everyone withdrew from the bedroom. I lay on the bed wishing I could be anywhere else—at the top of Mt. Everest in a blizzard, on a twenty-six hour decrepit school-bus ride through Guatemala, in the middle of a colorectal exam. But fantasizing of alternative nightmares wasn't going to get me an epidural any faster. I rolled off the bed and opened the door.

"I'm ready to go now," I said. David sprinted down the hall to find my just-in-case-though-we-surely-won't-need-it hospital-transport bag. Martha kneeled beside me and steered my feet into a pair of underpants and then pulled my least-favourite black maternity dress over my head. As I got dressed, Jade came back into the room to gather her things and stepped on the hand mirror Martha had left on the floor. The mirror shattered into a hundred tiny pieces as I reminded myself that I'm not superstitious, except that I am.

I took the steps one by one, leaning heavily on the banister. I could feel something dripping down my bare leg. As I stepped outside into the bright, hot midday sunshine, I immediately longed for my dark cave. David helped me into the back of our hot car where I immediately lay down and resumed my groaning. Rose drove and David sat up front with an arm reached back to pat me reassuringly.

It was a long ten-minute ride to the hospital during most of which I was sure I could feel a head pushing against my underpants. David wheeled me to the hospital lobby, the midwives tagging along behind us and Rose staying behind to park the cars. We rode the elevator to the fifth floor with several other passengers. I had never been on an elevator with a woman in labour and, from the looks on their faces, neither had they. My contractions were back-to-back by then and I was squirming and writhing and stiffening in my chair as though it were electrified. I didn't feel comfortable moaning and screaming and grunting in public, so I gritted my teeth and held it all in and the pain doubled. Soon, I reminded myself, I would get my epidural. Soon, soon, soon. It was 1:30 in the afternoon.

At the nurse's station, Jade quickly briefed the nurse-midwife while I did my silent contortions. A nurse wheeled me into a delivery room with my entourage close behind. I expected to find an anesthesiologist waiting for me in this room, epidural in hand. Instead there were forms to sign, hospital gowns to get into, fetal monitors to attach and an IV to stick in my arm.

A nurse came to my bedside waving her hospital tag and telling me that normally she wore two tags but that she had misplaced her other one and that if any hospital staff wearing fewer than two tags ever tried to take my baby, I shouldn't let them. Was this woman crazy? Why was she lecturing me about infant abduction when my baby wasn't even born yet? Couldn't she see that all I cared about was pain relief? Finally, she asked me if I wanted "something to make me feel better." Now we were getting somewhere.

"That's why we're here!" I was about to shriek, but decided

instead to nod appreciatively. She smiled approvingly. "The anesthesiologist is in surgery now. He'll take care of you as soon as he's out."

Say what? There was only one anesthesiologist for the whole maternity ward and he was in *surgery*? That was impossible. One of the reasons I had opted for home birth was because I knew how hard it would be for me to resist drugs where they were so readily available. Now, here I was, begging for anesthesia, and I would have to wait. I started to cry. I felt very, very sorry for myself. I was certain that my pain would never end and my baby would never be born.

David, Jade, and Martha stood around the bed comforting me, holding my hand and saying things I don't remember as the contractions thrashed and rocked me. Laurel rejoined us after her other mother finished birthing her baby.

At 3:15 p.m., the anesthesiologist made his appearance, a halo of light hovering over his head. "I will marry this man," I thought. He had me sit on the edge of the bed and lean forward against David while he pushed a gigantic needle into several spots on my back. The shots were painful, but within five minutes my contractions began to fade from awareness and before long I couldn't feel them at all. All I could feel was a heaviness in my legs, a tingling in my toes, and some pressure against my rectum where the baby's head was resting.

It was the purest and most profound relief of my life. Everything suddenly seemed quiet and peaceful, even as a mind-bogglingly large number of hospital staff bustled around the small room. I began smiling and cracking jokes. I began to feel like I wanted to stay in this bed for a long time, possibly forever. I had never felt better.

Then, Dr. Basu entered the room.

One of the worst aspects of transporting from a home birth to a hospital birth is that you don't get to have your own obstetrician, because most obstetricians will not agree to provide backup to midwives. Instead, you get whichever staff obstetrician is on duty that day. Sometimes, the staff doctor is perfectly fine. Sometimes, she's not.

Dr. Basu is a very short, squat woman with unruly black hair. She wore yellow eyeglasses with purple polka dots. She entered the room as though she had just washed for surgery, with her hands held up in the air and a mask over her mouth. Silently, a nurse dropped an apron over Dr. Basu's head and tied it behind her back. Another nurse handed Dr. Basu a pair of latex gloves as though on cue. I thought she was preparing to examine me, but instead she began interrogating the midwives in a low, mildly accented, but barely decipherable mumble. Why had they let me push for so long? Didn't they know the baby couldn't pass through with the cervical flap in its way? Couldn't they see how exhausted I was? Why hadn't they transported me sooner?

The midwives calmly tried to answer her accusations, but they were clearly getting riled. They were trying hard not to seem like uppity midwives while still protecting their client's right to choose how she wanted to give birth. Finally, still without laying a finger on or saying a word to me, Dr. Basu declared that I would need a C-section.

Laurel balked. "You can't determine that yet. She just got an epidural and she's going to rest and then push again." They continued sparring until Dr. Basu issued her final ultimatum, "I'll give her two hours to push and then we're doing a 'C.'"

At that point I felt unconcerned. I'd just rest a little longer, maybe have a snack or two, and then I'd push this baby out. Laurel came to my bedside looking grave. "It's kind of bad luck that you got Basu. We have pretty good relationships with all the OBs here, except for her. She *hates* midwives and she *hates* home births, and she *loves* Cesareans."

The hospital nurse, who was wearing a Tibetan headband and an ROTC recruiting button, confirmed Laurel's characterization of Dr. Basu, but added that Dr. Basu was highly skilled at performing C-sections. "She truly believes it's the safest way for a woman to give birth and she's done thousands of them, and believe me she knows what she's doing. I've seen her save a woman's uterus."

I pictured a uterus flying out of a woman's abdomen and Dr. Basu catching it in midair and placing it back inside her. Then I noticed that Laurel was holding my hand and looking directly into my eyes.

"Erica, you're not having a C-section. Absolutely not, no way."

"Of course not," I said, thinking back to my own ultimatum a few hours earlier, "I'm having an epidural or a C-section *now*." Or was it an epidural *and* a C-section? Anyway, it wasn't a moment I was proud of and I was happy to join Laurel in pretending I had never said it.

"But," Laurel continued, "this two-hour time limit is real. You need to start pushing again now. And I think you should get some Pitocin to get your contractions going strong again."

"What about the cervical flap?"

"Don't listen to her. You can push through the flap if it's even there still. It's probably gone by now."

As the nurse set up the Pitocin drip, Laurel explained how we would do things. Since I couldn't feel my contractions anymore, Laurel would monitor them on the computer screen and would tell me when to push.

"How will I know I'm pushing? I can't feel anything," I asked.

"It's hard, I know. But, lots of women have given birth this way. Your body knows what it has to do."

Once the Pitocin kicked in, what had been moderately uncomfortable rectal pressure became intensely horrible. It wasn't exactly pain, not the kind of pain I'd been in before, but it was one of the most unpleasant sensations I'd ever experienced. The more I pushed, the more this sensation intensified. I pushed and pushed, never sure of how hard I was actually pushing or how far off my timing was.

"Can I stand?" I asked, hoping to enlist gravity's support.

"No," said the nurse. "Not with an epidural."

"Can I have some water?"

"You can suck on this." She handed me a lollipop stick with a small wet sponge on one end. "You can't have anything more than that in case you have to have surgery."

"But I'm really, really thirsty," I said.

She shook her head apologetically.

"You're at maximum-strength Pitocin," she said. "Now's the time for some serious pushing."

I spent the next hour doing some serious pushing. I held on to a bar and pushed. I held on to some rolled up sheets while David and Rose gave resistance from the other end, and I pushed. I counted to five and went full strength for all five counts. Then I tried pushing for as long as I could, taking a quick breath and going again as long as I could, then again, three times before resting, so that I was pushing for the full duration of the contraction.

I wasn't wearing my glasses and couldn't see clearly the mirror at the foot of the bed. But, it was reported to me that the baby's head was clearly visible, that with each push it was descending, but at the end of each contraction it was receding. I could sense the excitement in the room during the peak of the contraction, the little gasps and "ohs" and "yeahs" and then the disappointed sighs as my pushing weakened and the head disappeared again. I made no further progress.

When Dr. Basu came back into the room, it occurred to me for the first time that I was going to have a C-section and I began to feel scared. She put her hand inside me and felt the baby's head, then began mumbling. Everyone seemed to understand what she was saying, albeit with difficulty, except for me. David translated her mumblings. "She says he's stuck under your pubic bone. She says he's big and his head's at an angle. She says he's not coming out vaginally."

"We can try an extraction. Do you want an extraction?" she asked.

"What did she say?" I tried to keep the annoyance out of my voice, aware that this woman might soon have me under her knife.

"Do you want to try a vacuum extraction?" David said.

The vacuum was one of the many interventions we had sought to avoid by planning a home birth. "Well, if it's either that or surgery, I guess I should try it."

The ROTC nurse handed Basu an impossibly wide rubber suction cup. Basu wedged it into me and said I could try it up to three times.

"And then what?" I asked. David shrugged.

"Now," said Basu, and someone slipped an oxygen mask over my face as I began pushing my guts out while Basu yanked on the other end of the suction cup. Nothing happened.

"Push now," said Basu. I pushed. Basu frowned. "What's going on here? Are you pushing or pulling?"

It was then that the people and things in the room began to swim. I looked in the mirror and saw a horde of people I didn't recognize looking very busily at something. When I came back to earth, David was shaking his head back and forth angrily. I later learned that, on the second attempt, the nurse had inserted the vacuum backward so it didn't suction properly. That was why Basu had asked if I was pushing or pulling.

I waited to be told to begin my third and final attempt. Basu said that she had never seen the vacuum work after the first try and she didn't expect this time to be the exception. I heard that.

"Push," she said. This was it, my last chance to birth my baby in something resembling the way I had intended to. I strained with all my might. I gave it everything I had and then I reached deep and gave it a little more. Then Basu said, "It's not working. I knew it wouldn't work."

The room began to swim again. I was floating away from my body, unaware if I was still pushing, vaguely wondering who all the people around me were. When I came back to my body, the vacuum was out of me, and the room was quiet and still.

"I guess I have no choice now, right?" I smiled weakly at Laurel. "I mean, this baby isn't coming out of me any other way, is it?"

"It doesn't seem like it," she said. "You and David should take a minute alone to talk it over though."

"Prep her," said Basu as she left the room. The nurses nodded and then said they would come back in two minutes. It was 7:30 p.m., I had been in active labour for seventeen hours, much of it in excruciating pain, and now my rectum felt like an enormous, bulging hemorrhoid. I hadn't eaten in more than twenty-four hours and had slept for only two of the past thirty-six hours.

A number of panicky thoughts swirled through my head. Was this baby really stuck or was I submitting to this Cesarean fanatic's bullying? Would surgery be a terrible, possibly fatal mistake, or would it deliver to me a perfectly healthy baby in a matter of minutes? Above all, would I be able to take a nap when it was over?

"I think if I push for another hundred hours this baby won't come out," I said.

"It's totally your decision," said David. "I support whatever you choose to do."

"But, is it really even a decision at this point? I mean, what else can I do?" "I know. You've done it all. You've done the home birth and the hospital birth and the baby's still not out."

"But, this is the worst thing, the thing that we most wanted to avoid. We've done every single thing we didn't want to do and now here's the worst of all."

"None of that matters, though, as long as you and the baby are okay in the end. Remember the last card?"

"Healthy mommy, healthy baby," we recited together.

"Don't be hard on yourself, you did all you could. I can't believe what you've been through."

"Yeah well…call in the nurses before my anus explodes."

The ROTC nurse shaved me with an electric razor, catheterized me and put a pale pink shower cap over my head. David was directed to put on scrubs and meet me in the operating room. I was transferred to an operating table and wheeled into a frigid, fluorescent, stainless steel furnished room with the look and feel of a morgue.

David, in aquamarine scrubs and shower cap, held my hand as I shivered in my thin gown. My arms were extended out from my sides and tethered down to little tray tables on either side of me. As the anesthesia kicked in, I began to shake violently and understood that the arm restraints kept me from flying off the table.

"That's a common reaction," said the anesthesiologist.

A blue curtain stretched across my naval so that I couldn't witness the surgery, couldn't witness my child being born. David held my hand and leaned out to the side to peak around the curtain at times. As for me, I was floating high above the operating table in a morphine stupor, barely aware of any of the things being done inside my body. Beneath a hazy scrim I could make out Basu's black curls bobbing as she strained to pry the baby out of my uterus using what David described as a large shoehorn.

Suddenly, the anaesthesiologist was holding a purple-red baby near my face. "You have a boy," he said and then began to move away.

"Wait, wait," I cried and he brought my son back for a quick kiss. Then, a team of nurses whisked him away and out of sight to perform a number of tasks that hospitals deem more important than laying a newborn baby down on his mother's chest.

As Basu sewed me up, I wasn't shaking anymore, but I was confused and miserable and extremely cold. It wasn't entirely clear to me that I had just given birth. I needed to see the baby again to believe in his existence. David had gone with the nurses so he could stay close to the baby and make sure they didn't start trying to vaccinate him or shoot him up with antibiotics, or who knew what else.

Twenty minutes later, I was wheeled into a recovery room where David was waiting, holding a white swaddled package with a tiny face peeking out. I loosened the swaddling and laid my baby down on my chest. He quickly latched on to my breast, his bright eyes staring up at me with a look of wonder and mild alarm.

Then, the nurse helped David give Liam his first bath in a tiny tub set on a stand underneath a warming lamp. David struggled to sponge the sticky birth goo off Liam's floppy limbs, practically doubled over to avoid banging his head on the heat lamp positioned a few feet above the tub, a comfortable distance for most nurses, but not for a six–foot-two-inch man. He was utterly silent and grim-faced as he went about his task, but began yelping when he realized that the heat lamp was singeing his hair and beginning to burn his scalp. By the time he finished bathing and swaddling the baby, he looked approximately sixteen years older.

My parents arrived just as David handed the recovery-room nurse a Tupperware container and asked her to bring us the placenta. She looked merely amused as she informed him that the placenta was a biohazard and that we would have to dispose of it according to instructions she would give him.

"That's okay," David said, waving away the instruction sheet, "we're going to eat it." The nurse walked out, shaking her head in mild amazement. She snorted, but only a little. This was Berkeley, California, after all, where placentas often followed new parents home. But eating it was new to this nurse.

If the nurse seemed a bit taken aback, my mother was utterly astonished. She looked from me to David to my father, her mouth hanging open and her eyes wild.

"You're not...he's kidding, right?" She finally addressed herself to me.

"David's read up on it; it's really nourishing," I said.

"But, but...it's...I mean, you've got to be kidding me," she said.

"Gorillas eat it. All mammals do except for humans," David explained.

"Gorillas eat their stools, too," she said.

The nurse came back and handed David the Tupperware. The dark mass of placenta was visible through the sides of the container.

"We need you to take it home and put it in the freezer," I said.

David handed her the container. She looked down at it as if holding a radioactive device, then handed it to my father whose initial look of disbelief hadn't worn off yet.

This is where I had hoped my birth story would end, with my baby safely in my arms, surrounded by beaming father, mortified grandparents, and joyful midwives and friends, the smell of burnt hair infusing the air. It was to have been the last card—healthy mommy, healthy baby, but our deck had a wild card.

On the fourth morning of our hospital stay, the pediatrician noted that Liam's skin tone had become yellow and ordered a blood test for jaundice. A nurse came and stuck a needle in Liam's heel, which he didn't seem to mind. A few hours later, the pediatrician came back to tell me that his bilirubin level was on the high side and that he would reorder the blood test for the next day.

When he left, I whipped out my packet of new-parent brochures in search of information about jaundice. Jaundice, I learned, was a surplus of dead red blood cells, more than the liver was able to flush out of the body. It was apparently common in newborns and usually went away by itself or with exposure to sunlight. In more serious cases, the baby would be placed under ultraviolet lights and wrapped in a "bili-blanket" until the bilirubin count normalized, usually after a day or two. I concluded that Liam's mild jaundice was nothing to be worried about and returned to more pressing considerations, such as whether I'd ever have a bowel movement again.

By the next morning, Liam's bilirubin count had spiked to eighteen and the pediatrician said treatment was now necessary. Liam was very yellow—even the whites of his eyes had turned into little yellow saucers. David and I decided to have a portable ultraviolet-light treatment station installed at home—I was going to be discharged that evening, and we wanted desperately to be at home with our new baby. Our pediatrician said she thought doing the treatment at home would be fine. David went home to meet the technicians who would set up the treatment station.

When the news came that Liam's count had hit a terrifying twenty-four, I was alone and promptly burst into tears. The nurse sat on the edge of my bed. "Are you still planning to do the treatment at home?" she asked.

"Well yeah, I mean, I want to get out of here," I sputtered.

She inhaled deeply and looked me straight in the eyes. "Has anyone really explained jaundice to you?"

"No, I mean, just what I've read." I gestured toward the stack of flimsy brochures filled with pictures of non-yellow babies.

"You need to understand the risks—if your son's levels don't go back down soon, there can be brain damage. In extreme cases, well…he could die." I cried harder, shattered by this news. She took both my hands in hers. "It's a very treatable disease; it responds very well to the lights. I know that you want to go home, and that you're completely exhausted, but here in the hospital, we're set up to handle the kind of problem your baby has. We can get the jaundice under control and keep a close eye on him. If you do this at home, you'll have a bili-blanket, but not the overhead lights, and there'll be no nurses to help you. It's your decision of course…"

I was so utterly confused and terrified I could barely breathe. Should I bring my baby home or did he need to be handled by highly trained professionals? My fear quickly dictated the answer and David was in full agreement. He turned the technicians away at the door and stayed home to take a nap.

After forty-eight grueling hours in the NICU, Liam was finally given a farewell bath. David and I watched in awe as the nurse easily handled his floppy limbs and succeeded in cleaning him without drowning him, or setting her hair on fire. We agreed that we would never be capable of performing such a feat.

We walked out of the hospital into a blazing summer day, seven days after Liam was born. I hadn't set foot outdoors since my short journey to the car during labour, and the burning hot sun felt alien and hostile. I wanted to get into my bedroom and pull down the shades. We spent an amazing amount of time getting Liam into the infant car seat. I was tense the whole way home, certain that another car would plow into us at any moment.

And then we were at home with our new baby. I was drugged, exhausted, and traumatized, but alive and with no permanent damage. Liam was sleepy and yellow, but alive and with no brain damage. Healthy mommy, healthy baby.

Spring Baby
by Bridget Lamp

Thursday, April 16, at 2:30 a.m., I was startled out of bed. Contractions are often described as your worst menstrual cramps times one hundred. A nine-month break from cramps during pregnancy helped me forget what they are like.

"Ah ha! This must be it," I thought.

In our birth class our instructor, Penny, suggested distracting yourself during labour; doing whatever you can to get your mind off of the process. My husband, Eldon, and I watched *The Daily Show* and *The Colbert Report* reruns online.

We rode it out until 4:30 a.m., and then set up the contraction timer on the computer. My contractions were fifteen minutes apart. Eldon suggested we get some sleep, but the bed was the last place I wanted to be. I sat on my yoga ball and leaned forward on the couch, dozing to save strength. As several intense contractions came and went, Eldon asked what he could do for me. A sweet offer, yet I couldn't think of anything. I needed to get into my own zone. I waited until 6:00 a.m. to call our doula, Elisabeth. Having a little one of her own, I figured she'd be up by then.

"Hello?" Elisabeth's voice was cheerful. She'd been expecting my call as I was eight days overdue.

"I think this is it!" I told her.

When she arrived we walked to the bakery for pastries and coffee. I breathed with my eyes closed between bites and sips. We continued to the pharmacy, a distance I thought was too far, to pick up last-minute items. From there we went to the tennis courts to collect balls for Mudsy, our dog. I leaned on Eldon, leaned on fences, and leaned on telephone poles as my contractions intensified.

"How about we go this way?" Elisabeth was pointing at one of the steeper hills. I reluctantly agreed. I had been working out three times a week as well as working a physically demanding job. But during these last two weeks, I had just enough energy for work and maybe one swim or yoga session.

Back at the house, Elisabeth suggested I do some Cat-Cow yoga poses. My pain worsened. I complained.

"This is not about managing your pain. This is about getting the baby to move down," she replied.

Thinking about women's stories of their babies not being in ideal positions, and of long, drawn-out labours, I continued my poses; Mudsy joined in, nudging his face into mine.

Around noon, I asked Eldon when I would start active labour.

"Uh, you're already there," he responded.

"Really?" I couldn't believe it. I thought this whole time I was still in pre-labour. What a relief.

I was starting to progress further and called Dr. Ruddy around 3:00 p.m. My contractions were four minutes apart. Since she was on call at the clinic until 7:00 p.m., she offered that we could come in before going to the hospital, but understood if we wanted "one-stop shopping."

I mulled it over: one car ride versus two car rides. More than one person involved versus consistency. Since our birth plan specified that I only wanted Dr. Ruddy to check my progress, and the clinic was more or less on the way, I opted to go there first.

We left the house at 5:00 p.m. Our neighbours were out enjoying the warm spring weather. Between contractions, I managed to gracefully get in the car. Sitting on his front porch, my next-door neighbour raised his glass of red wine as we drove off. All the way to the clinic I braced myself for potholes and hummed like a bee as I had learned in my yoga class. We ditched our car in the no parking zone, our hazards on. I walked into the clinic and everyone sprang to their feet. I declined a wheelchair and walked into the examining room, bypassing the scale I had been weighed on weekly throughout my pregnancy. I breathed through the contractions with Elisabeth's reassuring words. Dr. Ruddy checked me and I was at four centimetres.

"See you at the hospital," she said. "But, you'll have to go to triage first since a room isn't ready for you yet." At the hospital, I slow danced with Eldon all the way from the parking garage to triage.

"How's your pain?" were the first words out of the nurse's mouth.

"Manageable," I replied. "I'm planning to have a natural birth."

She smirked. As she started to find a space for us, another nurse interrupted her, "Your room is ready." We skipped triage altogether.

In our birthing suite, I tried the rocking chair. I found the most relief sitting on the yoga ball leaning forward onto the bed.

The contractions were increasing intensity and a few got away from me. Elisabeth encouraged the tiny voice in my head that would help me get back into my zone. The nurses were keeping an eye on the waves of my contractions, but the numbers on the screen were not in sync with the sensations I was feeling. I closed my eyes and ignored it.

Dr. Ruddy checked in with us. I was free to move about, but mostly stayed on my hands and knees on the bed. The contractions, as intense as they were, weren't as bad as the quivering in my legs. My muscles needed relief. I wanted to soak in the tub. The doctor checked my progress: seven centimetres. When the tub was ready, I stood up and there was a huge gush. "So that's what it feels like when your water breaks!"

On my way to the tub, I vomited. Everyone scrambled to catch it, but no one was successful. Dr. Ruddy said triumphantly, "Welcome to transition!"

Twenty minutes in the tub helped calm my muscles and I moved back to the bed on hands and knees riding out the waves of progress. My noises became more guttural. I couldn't control what my body was going through and I didn't fight it. I was primal, animal-like. My doula and the nurse didn't interfere, even though they knew I was starting to push. Then I asked for the doctor. Nonchalantly the nurse said, "Okay. We'll get her."

I was checked and fully effaced at nine and a half centimetres. Dr Ruddy told me to "blow through my power to push" until I was dilated that last half centimetre. We'd brought a delicate Japanese pinwheel made of bamboo and *washi* for just this purpose. I blew and blew, keeping the pinwheel in constant motion until the go-ahead to push was given. I squeezed Eldon's hands hard as I pushed lying on my side. I lost track of time and opened my eyes once in a while to read my doctor. Everything was fine, just slow and steady. I heard cheers of "Good job!" and comments about how much hair they could see. As the baby crowned I managed to catch a glimpse. After almost two hours of pushing, I curled around my belly for one last push and let out a yell of relief. Our baby was born! I could hear the nurses scrambling and the baby crying.

"What is it?" I asked Eldon.

"It's a boy!" He said with a huge smile on his face.

He was born at 1:17 a.m. on April 17, weighing 7 pounds, 11 ounces, and was 19.5 inches long. The nurses brought him to my chest. He was long and kind of skinny, and looked at me with big gray eyes full of wonder.

"Hello, Oliver!" I greeted my son.

Arlo's Birth
by Patty Villaseñor

It's five days past my estimated due date, I have a pregnancy-induced rash on my belly that has been keeping me awake for about a month, everyone is asking when the baby is due, my sister is calling me every day, my daughter, Téa, has decided to sleep in our bed and my husband, Yori, is hoping this baby will stay in a little longer so he can get some more work done. I'm grumpy and sleep deprived and this baby hasn't even been born yet!

I was relieved, to say the least, when my contractions finally started at about 3:00 a.m. By 4:30 a.m., after unsuccessfully trying to sleep through some of the pain, I told Yori that he shouldn't go to work that day. He was a little disappointed that this baby didn't understand his work deadline, but agreed.

By 8:00 a.m. while trying to get breakfast ready for Téa, I found that I had to stop quite often during contractions to focus. I tried to do the laundry to take my mind off of it, but I couldn't do that either. Téa was not very understanding of mom's tummy pains, and became pretty grouchy that I couldn't sit and read her a book and would not let her climb on my back. Things had progressed quite slowly with Téa's birth, so Yori and I thought we had loads of time. However, by 9:30 a.m. I told Yori to find someone to watch our daughter because we'd have to go to the hospital pretty soon. I don't think he took me very seriously, but by 9:35 a.m. I was barking at him to get on the phone to Téa's godparents because we had to go. He and I were both a little surprised by the speed at which things were progressing.

We dropped off Téa on the way to the hospital. I remember working on my breathing and trying to relax my eyebrows. Yori was trying to drive steady enough that I wouldn't criticize him for being dangerous.

The hospital took me right into the examination room, and to my surprise an old friend's mom was supposed to be the nurse examining me. This was a little awkward for both of us, so she quickly reassigned herself. I was thankful for that.

It turns out I was immediately ready to go to the delivery room, so the nurse called my doctor, and it was looking like this might progress fairly quickly. Or, so we thought.

By noon I was eight centimetres dilated and things had come to a standstill. I was hungry and thirsty and thought maybe some apple juice would help. My body, however, had decided that it didn't want any food or drink and I threw up the apple juice.

I was having an increasingly hard time keeping my mind focused and together during the contractions. Yori, the champion masseuse, had been massaging my lower back for quite a while with me impatiently giving him instructions. I was trying to go as far as I could before asking for an epidural. When nothing had progressed for an hour, I asked for one. It took about forty-five minutes before it was finally inserted by a student anesthesiologist—amazing what you'll allow in such pain.

After the epidural we were still at a standstill. So, we hung out and talked with our doctor and nurse. They were both wonderful and interesting, but it was starting to feel a little weird lying there in a gown, making conversation to pass the time during labour. The excitement had been dulled by the pain relief, and now it seemed like an oddly quiet waiting game.

When it was finally time to push, I thought, "This is it! Our baby is coming!" Apparently, our baby was enjoying its cozy space though, because more than an hour later there was still no sign of him, and the blood vessels in my face were feeling like they were starting to pop from the pushing. We had tried a few different positions, but things just weren't progressing.

Finally, I thought, "Why don't I just squat?" I wish this had occurred to me sooner, because in no time our baby's head started to show and the excitement built once again.

After that, all I can remember is seriously painful pressure; the pressure was immense. I can't imagine what that would have felt like without the epidural. Women are truly capable of unbelievable feats.

Just when Yori was beginning to feel resigned to being surrounded by women, our baby boy, Arlo, was finally born. He was 8.5 pounds of pure screaming joy.

Naila's Birth
by Avanya Manasseh

My daughter was born on the day that she was due, September 28, exactly thirty-eight weeks to the day after she was conceived. That was the only thing about her birth that went as planned.

My essentially perfect, thirty-eight-week, illness-free pregnancy had finally grown old, and my husband, Jahan, and I were ready to stop looking forward to Naila's arrival, and get started on the parenting phase of our lives.

There was no aspect of Naila's birth that was not meticulously planned; every moment was calculated with greater detail than the creation of a piece of fine art. Long before I became pregnant, I had chosen a midwife, and on the morning I saw two very clear pink lines while waiting breathlessly in the bathroom, I wasted no time in contacting Connie.

From the start, we loved planning Naila's birth with Connie. We were joyous to have found a professional, caring midwife who attended home births. We loved working with her month-by-month, planning out the big day. Jahan and I read books on home births, and scoffed at the idea of a hospital birth for our baby girl, who deserved the most natural, serene entry into the world. We spent the long months of pregnancy practicing

HypnoBirthing, a theory that involves learning about your body's birthing process and working with the sensations that occur, instead of fighting against them.

So with months of preparation behind us, I nervously told Jahan one Saturday that I believed the labour process had started. A cramping feeling came and went in the wavelike pattern that had been described to me so many times. True to our plans, we quietly went about our day, knowing that the best thing I could do was to stay as active and distracted as possible.

As planned, we picked up our friends for lunch to celebrate their recent engagement. With our huge secret between us, I welcomed the opportunity to focus on diamond rings and invitation ideas, sharing in the glow of the beginning of another new family and remembering fondly our own journey there just five years before.

We drove to the beach and leisurely ate lunch overlooking the ocean. I felt the waves inside me mirroring those I gazed out upon, and knew that something was happening within me. My little friend was soon on her way to meet mommy and daddy! We sipped our cool water, felt the ocean breeze brush our cheeks, and looked at one another slyly while I gorged myself on french fries.

Getting back into our car, I felt a warm pool suddenly form under me and realized that my water had broken! I turned to Jahan and our friends and nervously muttered that we had better hurry home.

Jahan looked at me in shock and asked, "What do we do?" Connie's training set in and I quickly pulled her number up in my cell phone and left a message. When she called right back, her calmness reassured me that no baby would be arriving on the way home, and that she would get ready and be on her way.

Jahan quickly dropped off our guests while I settled at home with my mom, figuring out how to sit on a towel and wondering when things would pick up. While I still felt contractions, I was in no real pain. My mom hurried around the house, washing towels and making sure all of our birthing supplies were ready.

During the next few hours, things slowly progressed. I went from giggling in my chair to rocking rhythmically back and forth in the birthing tub. "Relax, relax, release," was all I could think. My mind was completely clear of everything but those words, as I saw them circling my head again and again. My eyes were closed and I saw nothing on my eyelids. Everything was blank, waiting for my baby girl to make her mark on my life. Only from time to time was my focus interrupted to get antibiotics, or to try to eat something, as Connie so wisely forced nutrition and hydration during labour.

I was unaware of time, but realized eventually that darkness and sleep had fallen on the house. The only lights were in my bedroom, and inside of me waiting to come out. I saw Jahan's head bobbing and losing the fight against sleep as he sat in his chair next to my tub. I heard my mother in the hallway, lying down but ready and on guard. When Connie came to listen to the heartbeat I saw the sleep in her eyes, and slowly all this began to add up in my mind; it was late in the night. Connie told me to tell her if I felt the urge to push, but I never did. Slowly, I began to wonder why. Connie encouraged me to change positions to bring the baby down better, and I unhappily acquiesced. I could see the concern growing in Jahan's eyes as he watched me stay committed to our plan.

Hours later, Connie came to my side and told me she had called the doctor, and we had to go to the hospital. I saw the light coming through the closed curtains behind her head, and sadly acknowledged that this would not be the birth we had hoped for.

In one swift motion, that decision turned our whole course another way. Quickly, bags were gathered, clothes were found, and we were on our way to the hospital, a trip I never imagined making. Once we arrived I retreated into my silence again, knowing that once I started vocalizing the pain, without my last thread of focus, there would be no turning back.

As we were set up, I was told I would have Pitocin and an epidural. My body was too exhausted, I had to rest, and not enough progress was being made. I knew that if I resisted this, they would quickly order a Cesarean. The nurses told me I would probably have one anyway, and had my mom take all my jewellery from me. My mother, steady and calm, assured me again and again that it wouldn't happen. I could do it.

Finally, an epidural intact, Pitocin pumping through my veins, I rested. Later, I begged to have the epidural taken out. I hated the loss of control, the inability to feel my own body. While the nurses resisted, my doctor stood by me, and allowed it to be taken out.

So it was pumped full of chemicals that I pushed and pushed my 8-pound, 13-ounce beautiful Naila into our world, more than twenty-four hours after my water broke, more than thirty-six hours after my first gentle contractions. I screamed like every other labouring mother: no peaceful music, burning candles, or birthing tub. Rather, the doctor had to reach inside me and pull her head out while I screamed for all the world to hear.

Naila was asynclitic, a word I had never heard before in my life. Connie told my mother just a few hours into my labour that she suspected this was the case. Instead of simply coming down the birth canal head first, she did so while tilting her head off to the side. When she was born the huge cone on the side edge of her head confirmed Connie's early diagnosis.

From before she was born, Naila was someone we could never have been prepared for, though we didn't know it until after she was here. Each day she surprises us just as much as her first day in this world. Her birth was not what we hoped for, but she is so much more.

Shaking the Breathing Birthing Tree
by Sej Morrice

Of course, this story starts months before the actual event, but I will begin a few days before actually giving birth, when I started actively doing things to help induce the contractions. Monday evening I spent most of my prenatal yoga class weeping in a ball on my mat. I just felt so full. I was starting to think Tuesday might be the day, but when I only had a few contractions that evening, I just tried to relax and go to bed without too much anticipation or pressure.

I awoke Wednesday at 7:30 a.m. with some pretty good contractions and I stayed in bed resting, snoozing, and counting. After six contractions in a row, I called my friend who was attending our birth as the beginning of her hands-on doula training, and then my midwife just to check in. When she arrived a little after 11:00 a.m. she confirmed I was "a very soft four centimetres," and really in labour! I had thought that my contractions weren't long enough or close enough together, but she counted for me and told me they were about four to five minutes apart and up to one minute long. I guess I was already so into it that my brain wasn't working in normal time.

We started the final preparations of inflating the birthing tub in our bedroom and listened to "Shaking the Tree" by Peter

Gabriel.

For the next hour or so I laboured on my yoga mat on the dining-room floor. I mostly sat on my feet with my hands in front of me like a cat, or on hands and knees, making low "mmmmm" sounds and sort of tossing my head around to keep my face and shoulders loose through each contraction. My toddler even came to join me on the floor, getting into the same positions and making the same sounds, which was very sweet.

My labour was intensifying and I reminded myself of the Birth Affirmations my friends and I had hung in my bedroom during my Birth Room Blessing, things like: *welcome love; I claim my birthright for a wonderful birth; I am never alone, I have sisters throughout the world who are birthing their babies at the same time as me. I tune in to them and send them my love and reassurance*; and *right now, right now, right now* instead of *this sucks, this sucks, this sucks*. It worked marvelously. The more I stayed present to the birthing experience and the wisdom of my body, the easier it was.

Soon my neighbor came to pick up our son and I think that really helped me get to work. My legs and knees were getting sore from being in the same position all morning and someone suggested I try leaning on the couch, but I couldn't get comfortable so it was more frustrating than helpful. I then moved to our futon mattress on the floor in the living room and assumed a similar position to the one I had been in all morning, but this time I was supported by many pillows and could relax more.

Our apprentice midwife, spent some time with her hands resting on my back. It had to be a very specific place just above my lower back and I would occasionally reach around to move her hands a tiny bit. She graciously followed my requests. Then my husband came and took over with his hands on my back and was also willing to do just as I asked. I had thought I'd want lots of pressure on my lower back like I did during labour with my first child, and my husband and I had been practicing that, but I wasn't having back labour this time. Instead, I just needed a calm supportive presence to keep me grounded.

During my labour I felt like I was a channel for all the energy in the universe, and also that I could read other people's energy, or tune it out if needed: my doula was infuriatingly calm, my midwife was trying so hard to be respectful and out of the way that I actually picked up on her a little more, the assistant midwife was calm and mellow, my neighbor was almost vibrating with excitement and positive energy, and my husband was bouncing off the walls, running around preparing stuff until I needed him and then just seamlessly meshing with me when I needed him— he was absolutely perfect.

After the futon, my husband and I tried labouring standing up, which I didn't like, but it did help to move labour along and bring the baby down. It was then that I started really thinking about the birth tub. It sounded great and I had been looking forward to it for all these months, but I didn't want to get in too soon because if labour slowed down, as it can in water, I'd have to get right back out. We checked with midwife and she gave me the go-ahead to get in.

The spot I chose for my birth tub was in our second-story bedroom, near a window looking out at a large apple tree. This tree is important to me because buried underneath it are the ashes of my parents as well as the little ball of cells I miscarried a year ago; the apples from the tree nourish my family and friends each autumn. On the wall of the room were paintings and images of women that felt sweet and powerful to me.

I was listening to "Breaths" by Sweet Honey in the Rock, the most beautiful and perfect song for this time.

I was feeling my grandmother's and mother's spirits with me and I cried and rejoiced to have them so close.

Sometime around 1:00 p.m., our son was brought home for his nap, and by the time he got up, I had been in the birth tub for about half an hour. When I first got in it was a bit disconcerting; although the inflated bottom and sides were super-comfy, the floating feeling wasn't, and it took awhile to get my bearings and to find a position to labour in. I wanted to be on all fours with my face down in the water, which of course didn't work very well, and my midwife reminded me that a sideways or bottom-down position would help the baby move down as well. I ended up on my side with my face half in the water. This is how my boy found me at 2:30 p.m. after waking up, and he thought it was pretty funny that I was blowing bubbles in a bathtub in "Mama-Papa Room." Shortly after he left again for the neighbor's.

After about an hour of labouring in the tub by myself, with the midwives quietly keeping me company, I asked to have my husband with me in the tub and we were left alone to labour together. We also changed music, to a chant CD by Robert Gass that was a perfectly peaceful backdrop for this quiet, intense time. This was the beginning of the hardest and most wonderful part of the whole day. My husband was completely present and did everything I needed. He sat cross-legged behind me as I lay curled up on my left side in his lap, and he brought his left hand under me and held it over my heart, which perfectly calmed me and held me in the grace and serenity I needed so much.

At about 3:40 p.m., several things happened, either all at once or in quick succession: the nature of the contractions changed, from pressure across my lower belly to wrapping around my sides and back; I no longer got a real break between contractions; and I felt my whole pelvis start to open up. The energy I'd felt as a ball in my belly transformed into a two-way stream going all the way through me and I noticed the sounds that were being made—by me, of course, but at the time I didn't think of it that way—were higher and louder, which brought the midwives back. I also felt like giving up and throwing up.

I said this last part out loud, expecting someone to tell me I was in transition, but instead my husband said, "You can do this, you *are* doing this, you're doing so well." So I decided to act like I was in transition anyway. I focused on opening and releasing my pelvis and I just let everything go. It was like falling into a whiteout abyss. I was overtaken by the immense, intense, all-consuming power of birth.

I suspected the urge to push, and said out loud, "Push!"

One of the midwives asked if I was asking to have my husband push on my back. But I said, "No, *push!*"

I got the go ahead to push if I really needed to. At that point there was no decision to be made as my body was just doing it, the way it was meant to be, the way it's been happening to women across time. At about 3:50 p.m., one huge, yelling push barreled through my whole being and suddenly the baby's head was right there and my water broke with meconium everywhere.

"Get out of the tub now," I was told. We'd planned to birth in the water, but meconium, the baby's first poop, can be a sign of fetal distress. The safest thing was for me to get out of the water right away. I was totally willing to comply but could not figure out how to get out, or where to go. My husband jumped out and helped me up. When I stepped out I really thought for a second I was going to give birth standing on a towel-covered tarp in the middle of our bedroom, which would have been totally fine.

Fortunately, the bed had been prepared and I was helped up onto it. My husband sat behind me, holding me up and supporting me. I pushed one more time and the baby's head was crowning. I reached down and touched the slippery head as I was told to wait. There was that timeless feeling again as we waited for the next contraction and then it overcame me without a thought and my beautiful baby was born all at once into the midwife's hands, and onto our bed where he was first dreamed of all those long months ago.

I had hoped to have a few moments with my child before I knew if it was a boy or a girl, but he was born so quickly, right there in front of me, that I immediately said, "It's a boy!"

His cord was so short that it detached from the placenta when he was born, so the midwife had my husband cut it right away. As soon as our baby was nursing, I had to birth the placenta, too.

Our son was born at 4:05 p.m., weighing 9 pounds, measuring 20.5 inches long, and his head was 15 inches around; one of the largest our midwife had ever seen! A week after our baby's birth, I felt better than I did a month after our older son was born in the hospital, drug- and intervention-free. In some ways I felt better than I ever had now that our family was complete.

Weirdness in my Nether-Regions
by Lindsey Gregg

"Your delivery was…just…weird," said my midwife about one week after our baby was born.

Weird.

A description I found paradoxically frustrating and a little bit comforting as I sought an explanation—of sorts—to make sense of the many zigs and zags our delivery path took over four days starting on an April Saturday. Our baby finally arrived Tuesday morning.

Yes, yes, the birth experience is unpredictable and Birth Plans go according to plan infrequently at best. They should be renamed Birth Plans of False Hope. Or Birth Buckshot. Or Some Random Ideas You Have Bothered Putting Stock In For The Past 40 Weeks. I don't resent a Birth Plan, per se. I am sure they help women stay calmer and more focused than having no personal preference for her delivery experience. They are just really inaccurately named.

But now that I had a bouncing baby I wanted my midwife to help me make a summary of the experience. I wanted *learnings* so if we have a second child I won't feel so desperately wrecked for eight days following the magical act of delivering a baby. I wanted her to say, with reassurance, "Well, it turns out your extra-long torso means you had to push harder and longer than we thought and we didn't coach you properly in the first couple of hours to do so. Now we know for next time." Or something. Anything.

But instead I got a fragmented, puzzled, "weird."

So perhaps my catharsis will be in the act of writing this story. Our story. Like tying a weird little bow around our weird little family.

Forty-one weeks of pregnancy brought me no more discomfort than prenatal carpal tunnel which slowly trickled numbness into my middle fingers at about month six and spread through my hands until well after delivery. It took about two months to completely fade away postnatal, which made the closing of tiny sleeper and onesie snaps rather annoying for lack of feeling in my fingertips. I slept in wrist braces. It was irritating, but I got off lightly given the complications that often come with "geriatric" moms (I was 36 for my first child).

We are Canadians living in the Netherlands, which is a great country in which to deliver babies. It has a midwife system that may be unparalleled globally, and each mother gets one whole week of FULL TIME, AT HOME nursing from a postnatal specialist who teaches you how to breast feed, bathe junior, charts healing and will even make you a meal or two and do some basic cleaning. It is part of the Dutch public health system to give babies and moms the best start possible. Amazing.

Given all of this, our particular Birth Buckshot read something like this:

- Labour at home as long as possible, and then go to the birthing ward at the Dutch hospital (two blocks from our home).

- Reserve the "penthouse" birthing room complete with huge

tub, stereo system and amazing view of Den Haag.

- No epidural, but I am not being a hero. It's ok if I change my mind.

- Must ask my permission for an episiotomy (we had been told that they tend to give them in the Netherlands).

- Must ask my permission to conduct other interventions.

- Baby on breast immediately following delivery (this is also Dutch protocol with healthy babies).

- Husband Josh will cut the umbilical cord.

- Please put placenta in the container provided for processing into capsules.

Looking at this list, we got 3 out of 8, so I am wondering why it felt so chaotic…Anyway, here goes:

Tuesday
My due date came and went.

Thursday
I did acupuncture and had a halfhearted membrane sweep to get things moving. I was a centimeter dilated!

Saturday
One of the four midwives from our practice came by for a second membrane sweep.

"You're a centimetre dilated. That's a good sign."

OK, still a centimetre, so no change in two days. But it can change at any minute and at least we're heading in the right direction.

While eating dinner I started to get my first pangs of

contractions. My waves came in about every 15 minutes from 7:00 p.m. until 4:00 a.m. and then quit altogether. I slept in 15 minute intervals between squeezes and then passed out from 4:00 a.m. to 8:00 a.m. Disappointment reigned when I woke.

"Damn. One sleepless night for nothing," I said.

"But it's starting!" said hubs.

True.

Sunday

We went to the market with my parents who were here from Canada. Walked around, feeling good.

At 7:00 p.m. during dinner it started again.

"OOOH, I hope this is it!"

And it was!

No it wasn't.

From 7:00 p.m. until 6:00 a.m. my contractions gradually picked up from 20 minute to six minute intervals. We were certain we would be calling the midwife within the hour when they started receding back up to 15 minutes where they stayed. And stayed. And stayed.

"What the hell!?" I cried.

"It'll be ok," said hubs. "I'm sure you're making progress.

Monday

I wasn't.

That morning, another midwife came by for an exam and broke the news, "You're still at 1cm," she said.

Two sleepless nights for nothing.

I cried.

"It's like your uterus and your cervix are not communicating," she explained. Then she looked closely at my face, "Ya, you're not *there* yet. Women who are almost giving birth are in this crazy zone. You're not in that zone yet, not even close."

"So what do we do?" asked hubs.

"You wait," said midwife with a shrug. She was a bit of a rookie, and in hindsight perhaps not the best match for my personality. Waiting sucked, but would have been easier if she had said, "This happens sometimes. You need to give your body a chance to respond. You need to force yourself to relax." Or something. Anything.

This worried me. I was unable to rest and starting to feel desperate and hysterical. I was going to labour unproductively for the rest of my life, I was certain. This was my lot.

"She hasn't slept in two days and she hasn't even started dilating," said hubs. "If this goes on and on she won't have any energy to push. She already doesn't want to eat…"

Words like "induction", "balloon", "oxytocin", "sedation to rest", "book appointment with the doctor in the hospital" bounced around. She made a few calls.

"So, they won't induce you at the hospital today. Only after an examination from the hospital doctor, and the first appointment for that is 11:00 a.m. tomorrow. Then they might put you on a balloon or Pitocin, but they only do that in the evenings, so you have to wait anyway."

Seriously? I had to wait AT LEAST 36 more hours just to be induced? I was incredulous. Furious.

"What do we do until then? She needs to get some rest somehow."

"Well, tonight at 10:00 p.m. you can go in and they will give you a sedative with a bit of sleep aid in it to help you rest. It will last five hours. You won't actually be asleep, you will still feel the contractions, but it will help you rest. It will not harm the baby. You can then have your appointment with the doctor at 11am. Don't bother bringing your hospital bag. Oh, and your husband cannot stay over with you."

"Like hell I'm not," whispered Josh beside me.

That was the plan.

We arrived at the hospital that night with toothbrushes in our pockets and nothing more. My parents were on dog duty at our house with their fingers crossed.

Into a tiny "sedation room" we went. I was put on a heart monitor for 30 minutes, examined again with a 2cm result and then viciously stabbed in the thigh with a needle. Josh managed to wheedle a bed out of one of the nurses instead of being sent home (that is actually the feat of the entire experience, given how "This is not possible" is the mainstay of Dutch communication when you ask for any favours to be done that are outside of protocol). It was 10:30 p.m. and I was drifting into an opiate haze.

And then waking for a contraction. Ouch.

And then drifting.

And waking. Ouch.

Drift.

Contract. Ouch.

Drift.

Tuesday

"I think my water just broke." Ouch.

Drift.

"What if I missed my window for an epidural?" Ouch.

Drift.

"Seriously. Call the nurse." Ouch.

Drift.

My poor sober self was fighting to emerge prematurely from the sedation. I was told to expect to be under until about 4 a.m. It was 12:30 a.m.

The nurse came in while I was trying to find words through the haze.

"Ok, yes, this isn't urine, but it is probably just your first waters membrane as there isn't too much liquid. I will call your midwife," she said.

More people and the rookie midwife arrived and I was examined again.

"WOW! You've gone from 2cm to 8cm in two hours! It looks like we are going to have a baby soon!!"

Fuck, like THIS?? I felt high as a kite. How the hell can I breathe through contractions and meditate and push when I can barely utter a coherent sentence. I am not at the top of my game. I am not even in the game. I am getting high in the park with my friends when I am supposed to be across town at the game. No, no no…

"I need to push."

"You DO?"

"Ya, I need to push."

And so I pushed as unproductively as expected given my state of mind and body. I pushed and walked and stood and pushed and could not get a feeling for it no matter which position I tried. My midwife watched and provided a few tips to help but it wasn't landing. It was frustrating. Hours passed.

My midwife said to me, "I think we will have to use Pitocin to strengthen your contractions. This baby is not coming down."

In the Dutch system this is called "going medical". It means your care is transferred from the midwife to the doctor in the hospital and dreams of light touch childbirth are gone. I was going medical. I didn't really care anymore.

Forty-five minutes later in walked a new doctor. She was energetic and looked me in the eye and took control. I liked her immediately. But she took her bloody time getting here.

"This baby is face up," she said right away. No wonder I was having trouble moving it down.

"We are going to put you on a Pitocin IV. It will take 40 minutes to take effect. Try to not push during this time."

(Side note: As I write this, my baby is 6.5 months old. In my entire pregnancy and motherhood experience there are two things I can say with conviction that I hate. The first is how I felt when I was told "Try to not push." It was a mixture of helplessness, desperation, indignation, and disbelief. Try to not push. Ha. Try to not breathe. The second is breast pumping. I find it demoralizing).

And so I pushed with futility with my midwife and hubs coaching. It was not great.

Forty minutes later Dr. Jolande jumped in.

"Ok, Lindsey. Listen to me. Stop making noise. You need to redirect that energy to pushing. You will push three times with each contraction. Each time for twenty seconds. This will hurt like hell but you can do it. Take a deep breath quickly between your pushes and do not let go."

And we did. And the baby crowned!

And receded.

And crowned.

And receded.

On and on and on. Hours passed. I ripped out my IV trying. They had to move it to the other arm. I pushed and pushed.

"I think we will have to use the vacuum. The baby's heart rate is starting to respond. It has been inside for a long time. I will call the gynecologist at home to come in."

I was destroyed. It was 5:00 a.m. and I had been pushing for more than four hours and I thought we were almost finished. I looked at hubs, "I cannot do this. I cannot," I pleaded. "I cannot wait another 40 minutes for a doctor to show up to get this baby out. I cannot do this." I was silently begging someone to take the responsibility off my shoulders and say the word Cesarean.

Dr. Jolande left the room and my midwife looked at me.

"Lindsey, you are so, so, so close. We will have this baby out before the gynecologist even gets here. You can do it," she said.

At some time earlier hubs had called my parents to bring my hospital bag and they were in the waiting room at the end of the hall. All had been silent for hours, but when they saw what looked like 10 people surrounding a bed with me being rushed down the hall into a bigger room they thought I was headed for surgery. Luckily it was just a venue change. This room had stirrups and I could get leverage to push. I dug deep.

And I pushed and pushed and pushed and pushed and pushed.

"I see dark hair!" a chorus sounded from my vagina.

"That's not dark!" said hubs, "That's ginger!"

The gynecologist arrived in a record 15 minutes. I was injected with a local anesthetic "in case" I needed an episiotomy. They didn't ask, they just went ahead and cut me. It was necessary for the vacuum. It was a big cut. I felt the warm blood run over my bum. I didn't really care anymore.

More things were inserted inside me. I pushed. They did the tiniest of vacuums and my baby's head was out!

One more push and its body was there!

And then our baby was on my chest.

I could hardly believe it. I didn't believe it. I just looked at Josh who was smiling through tears. I was frozen from feeling anything. I was on duty. I was busy. I was pushing. I was digging deep, concentrating. I was trying so, so, so hard.

"It's here, Linds, it's here." Deep breath.

Our baby was two minutes old before we even checked its gender.

A boy. I knew it!

At five minutes old he was suckling at my left breast, which would become his favourite. When he is older we will embarrass him by telling him he "loved Lefty".

At ten minutes old he had a name, paying homage to Josh's father who had died of lung cancer when I was three months pregnant.

At 40 minutes old he met his grandma and grandpa, his Nanny and Papa.

Our son was born at 6:08 a.m. He was 3.875kg. He was 51cm long. His APGAR score was 10. We had a healthy baby.

The single proud moment I will allow myself in this ever-so humbling experience is remembering the words from the medical student who was also on duty, assisting my delivery. She is also named Jolande. When it was all over and I was stitched up, she stood beside me at the bed, looked at me and said with so much emotion in her young eyes, "I want to tell you that you are an inspiration to me. I want you to know this."

My recovery was tough for a myriad of reasons. I had all the damage that you can imagine from pushing a face-up baby for so long. But it was straight-forward healing, no complications.

Eight days later I looked at my midwife who had dubbed my labour "weird". Considering she had hundreds of words to choose from, and considering that our son had skyrocketed past his birth weight and I had managed a poop or two, her appraisal was probably accurate as far as she was concerned.

And as I write this, I am watching my hilarious boy launching himself up and down in a Jolly Jumper. He was born to laugh with dimple adorned cheeks, his momma's complexion and hair, a curious mind and his father's eyes. I hope he grows up as resiliently as he entered the world, needing only the smallest of sucks from the vacuums of life to help him when he needs it. And I suppose weird is pretty damn good.

There's No Place like Home
by Lisa Apligian

Our first child was born at home, in our one-bedroom apartment in the 18th arrondissement of Paris. Epidural capital of the world, the doctors thought I was totally insane for wanting to do this "on my own" and birth naturally. I was basically laughed at when I told my doctor that I didn't want an epidural. He informed me with a smirk on his face that I had to meet with the anesthesiologist regardless. Little did they know, I was planning, and ended up having, a home birth. My labour started at 1:00 a.m., and six hours later, at 7:00 a.m., my first child was born. That experience laid the foundation for my subsequent birth.

My husband and I had been living in Paris for four years when we decided it was time for a change. So midway through our fifth year, as we began the relocating process, we were happy to learn by way of a home-pregnancy test that we had indeed conceived! A few weeks into the pregnancy, I remember sitting by the kitchen window desperate for sunlight on yet another cold, gray, rainy, dreary Parisian day, extremely exhausted, extremely tired, extremely nauseous, much more so than the first time. I was still nursing my two and a half year old, so I attributed these extremes as too much for my body to be nursing while pregnant.

From my first birth experience, I learned what it truly meant to "birth from within," to trust and listen to my body, my intuition, and my instincts. I was confident that I was making a connection with the life growing inside of me, just as I had done with my first child, so my first doctor's appointment wasn't until I was thirteen weeks along. I didn't think anything of it when she heard a heartbeat about 2 inches apart from another heartbeat. Since our appointment was all in French and I hadn't learned the word "*les jumeaux*" yet, I know I missed a few things. I was sent to get an *échographie* (ultrasound) right away, two days after that first appointment. My husband, our little boy, and I went to the appointment and were sitting in the examination room merrily chatting, when the contents of my uterus were displayed on a big screen for all of us to see. My husband and I looked at each other thinking the same thing, "Isn't this interesting new mirror-image technology?" Hmm. It had been a few years, we did switch doctors, and this lady did seem to have newer equipment. Neither of us thought anything of it. "*Il y en a deux.*" Huh? We understood that: "there are two." There are two what? "*Des jumeaux*," "Two babies, twins." I was told to quit my job immediately and to stay off my feet.

From April to September, we packed up our apartment in Paris, shipped or sold our stuff, closed our accounts in France, did some travelling to Italy, Croatia, the Loire Valley in France, Spain, and then moved back to the good ole U.S.A. We bought a house, lived in four different places during the four weeks we were waiting for our house to close, furnished the house thanks to craigslist and garage sales, my husband painted a few rooms, we unpacked our storage unit, bought two cars, re-established ourselves as U.S. residents, my husband started a new job, and oh, yes, we interviewed and selected our midwives!

Finally, we were starting to settle in our new home, but we still hadn't received our shipment from France—more than fifty boxes including most of our baby things. It had taken fourteen weeks when it should have taken six to eight weeks, so needless to say, I was a bit frustrated with the movers. I just kept telling my babies to stay put! And they listened. Finally, our shipment arrived. I unpacked and sorted through twenty-five boxes and started to feel like everything was falling in place. It was then that I talked to Aidan, Twin A, and told him that he could now get ready. He was the bigger of the two, the one who would be born first. And he didn't hesitate.

The next day I kissed my husband before he left for work and we both commented that, "Today could be the day." I had started to feel some mild contractions the evening before, so we knew the time was drawing near. After he left, I was determined to get as much unpacking done as possible. I knew that I would not want to do anything, especially unpacking, after the babies were born. Two babies on their way, a three-and-a-half-year old, and no help except for my husband motivated me to unpack fourteen more boxes before leaving for the chiropractor with my little boy. It was there that I began having stronger contractions. She gave me an adjustment while my three year old played with some of the office toys and then sent me on my merry way. I arrived home at 12:15 p.m. and immediately started having strong, regular contractions. My water didn't break, nor did I lose my mucous plug like I had the first time by this stage in labour, but I just had a feeling that this was it.

I called and updated my husband, asking him to come home, but to stop at Home Depot on the way to get a new hose so we could fill up the little swimming pool we had for use during labour. I then called my midwife and talked to her for a bit about the contractions. She offered to come over, but I wanted to wait and ride them out on my own.

Around 1:30 my sweet husband arrived with a new hose, and started trying—without success—to blow up the pool with a foot pump. He didn't know what to do and was in a bit of a panic. I told him to try a hairdryer, but that didn't work either. We needed something with more power. He was clearly frustrated. We talked about our options and I still really wanted to try to get the pool blown up as I was in some serious labour pain. So, he ran over to our neighbour and asked to borrow a shop vac. She thought he was totally crazy asking for this in the middle of the week, in the middle of the day, acting weird and with his nice clothes on. "Um, no, but you can go to Home Depot and get one," was her response. He didn't explain. We couldn't blow up the pool, but at this point, I was pretty much done caring about the pool as I just needed him to check on our son and get things ready for the birth.

My husband put on an all-time favourite movie, *Peter Pan*, for our little boy to watch upstairs in our townhome, as I yelled through the contractions. I went into the bathroom, held on to the towel holder, opened my mouth and let the pain trample over my vocal chords. Then I'd walk, and walk, and walk until the next one and do the same thing, all while my husband was running around frantically trying to get everything ready. He laid down a tarp we had used for painting and put a couple of towels over it for me to rest on and push, and he managed to find the supply box for the midwives. I asked him to take off my clothes as I was ready to push. Just then one of the midwives arrived. Thank goodness we at least had a decent fence in our backyard because we still hadn't gotten around to hanging curtains. Oops!

I started pushing. "*Aaahhh!* He's coming, he's coming!" I knew something was making its way down, of course thinking all the while it was a baby, so happy that this was it—what else could it be? But low and behold, my midwife burst my bubble.

"No, it's just your sac of water." *What?* All that work just for a freaking sac of water? Argh. I guess it did come out a bit quick to be a baby. Later she told me that I birthed my sac intact because I had eaten so well and all that protein had made the sac very strong. But, I had no time to ponder this because Traveller Number One was on his way.

Twin A made his way pretty quickly, though in the moment it seemed like forever. I had been daunted by the option of catching my first born and regrettably passed up the chance. I didn't want to miss out again, so I kept reaching down, feeling for my little baby, searching for his head, when finally I felt it. It was just enough to give me that added bit of strength to push, push, *push* him out. I was so amazed to have caught him. I did it! I was just so proud and had such a reward in my hands. But, there was still another baby inside me, so I just sat there wondering what to do with Twin A. I really didn't know. I wanted to hold him and bring him to my chest, but his cord was too short, and I wasn't sure about the time frame for the next one in waiting. My midwife helped me rest him on my stomach as I held him with amazement and bewilderment. Only a few minutes later my midwife gave me the scissors to cut his cord, because the second baby was ready. So not only did I catch my baby, I cut his cord too!

After I cut the cord of Twin A, I gave him to his Daddy to hold while I worked on the second twin. Nine minutes after his brother paved the way, Twin B shot out so fast and slippery that I just couldn't catch him! I didn't have to do much pushing for him since he was a little smaller. He was still in the caul, so upon entry to the plastic tarp, my midwife grabbed hold of him, tore open the sac, pulled him out, and gave him to me. He was such a pistol, and still is!

My babies were born on October 3, nine minutes apart, the first at 3:45 weighing 6 pounds, 14 ounces, and the second at 3:54 weighing 6 pounds, 4 ounces. In numerology these are the numbers representing Truth and Trinity.

The second midwife arrived after travelling a great distance in Washington, D.C. traffic, very disappointed that she missed the excitement, but she immediately sat with me and got caught up. We left the cord attached to Twin B until my placenta was born, about twenty minutes later. I was not allowed to sit up until the placenta made its exit to avoid complications, mainly hemorrhaging. Birthing the placenta on my back was quite painful. It was definitely not as easy as birthing it upright, as I had done with my first child.

When Twin B's cord stopped pulsing, I cut that one, too. My midwives sorted through the placenta to make sure everything was intact and to see just how the two sacs had fused together to make one big placenta. I imagine that was a gold mine for them!

I continued to lie down and was given both babies, one in

each arm. That was very strange. I didn't have an extra hand to help a baby to a breast and really didn't know what to do. How do I adjust their heads or my arms, or feel their hands or their toes? I think everyone noticed how uncomfortable I looked and helped me get the babies nursing. Twin B had no problem suckling. He found the nipple right away, kind of sniffed it out. But, I needed quite a bit of help with Twin A to get him latched. That was so awkward I can't even tell you. My husband ended up helping me regularly for the first week and learned more than he ever wanted to know about breastfeeding, but boy did he get brownie points for that!

My midwife-in-training arrived while I was recovering and spoon fed me some soup. She was so gentle and nurturing, just exactly what I needed at that moment. Her help gave me the strength to crawl to the bathroom, just down the hall, a very momentous feat considering all that I had just done. I was very appreciative that my midwives escorted me every step of the way and was highly impressed with the amount of caution and care they gave me. After the birth, I felt much weaker than the first time, not realizing that losing 13 pounds of baby and twice as much placenta and fluids would really make that much of a difference. It took four days before I could climb down the stairs in our townhome to relax on the main level. My husband was amazing: he took care of me, cooked and brought me food, took care of the house and also our eldest child. He took two weeks off work to help me get up and going, helping me prepare to handle all three kids on my own full time.

I look back and am so thankful that I was able to birth all of my children at home. Birthing at home allowed me to tap into a strength I never knew I had, to delve into the most inner part of my being, and trust myself, my babies, and a higher power so completely. If you would have told me five or six years ago that I would have not one, but two home births, one of which was a twin birth, I would have told you that you were out of your mind. But, it was absolutely without a doubt the best place for me to bring life into the world. There's no place like home.

Acknowledgments

Thank you to Lisa Webb for appearing out of nowhere in a whirlwind of inspiration and showing me the way forward. I am so grateful for your example.

And to the team of creative women who contributed invaluably to the production of this book. I literally could not have done it without you.

Finally, thank you to all the writers/mothers who have sent us their birth stories since the first call went out years ago. We feel so blessed to have had you share them with us.

About the Contributors

Birth Writes brings together a gloriously varied group of talented writers who come from all walks of life. Among them are professional writers, gardeners, activists, teachers, doctors... The list goes on, but they all share one thing in common: They have a birth story to tell.

For more information:
www.livewithpositivity.com/books

About the Editors

Carole Monnier Clark, a mother of two beautiful girls, graduated with a Bachelors in English Literature as a result of her undying belief that life is shared through storytelling. Since then, she has travelled the world as a student, and now as a family, trying to piece together her own tale of life experiences. Recently, one of her stories about living as an expat appeared in the anthology *Once Upon an Expat*. She also writes about her other passion, Sophrology, with articles appearing in magazines in France and Bali. This book represents the denouement of just one of her many projects, who are still in the early stages of their rising action, in the midst of their climax, or satisfyingly cresting towards falling action and exist under the umbrella of Inner Roads Sophrology.

As a writer, Sophrologist, and now publisher, she has become certain that human experience is made richer by sharing in each other's stories.

www.livewithpositivity.com

Chelsie Anderson is a trained birth doula, professional organic gardener, and mom to 3 beautiful souls; Mali, Kale and Cohen. She is the owner and operator of Chelsie's Garden Soil-utions in Calgary, Alberta. Articles about her gardening adventures have been featured in local newspapers, and she actively contributes to various blogs. When she's not in the garden, she speaks publicly about her vast organic gardening knowledge and tweets about it @ChelsieSquared

During her pregnancies, Chelsie found that she had an insatiable appetite for birth stories, and with Ina May Gaskins books more or less ingrained in her memory, and with only one story being published by the local birth mag each quarter, she found there just weren't enough digestible stories available. Her wish is that through reading this compilation, women will have access to a range of modern birthing wisdom, as the sharing of a story is the most powerful way to support, nurture and prepare future moms for their own adventures in childbearing.

Made in the USA
Charleston, SC
20 January 2017